The Mystery of Hypertension

The Mystery of Hypertension

Hong Son Cheung

Library of Congress Control Number: 2008909382
ISBN: Hardcover   978-1-4363-7898-7
                 Softcover   978-1-4363-7897-0

To order additional copies of this book, contact:
Xlibris Corporation
1-888-795-4274
www.Xlibris.com
Orders@Xlibris.com
53094

Contents

To my dearest mother,

Mme. Lee Tsing Chin

to remember her for imparting her cultural education
in our life.

Also to my dearest father,

Cheung Mo Liang

To my dearest brother,

Mr. Christopher Cheung Hing Hung

to thank him for supporting our family in the earlier
time of our life

Also to my two dearest sons,

Noland and Alvin Cheung

Acknowledgment

I would like to thank those who supported me in writing this book. In alphabetical order, they were Alvin Cheung, Christopher Cheung, Noland Cheung, and Samuel Cheung.

I also would like to thank those who revised this book or other issues with all kind of suggestions. They were Alvin Cheung and Noland Cheung.

Foreword

I first met my teacher Hong S. Cheung in junior high at Chung Hwa Middle School, Brunei Town (now Bandar Seri Begawan), about forty years ago. Soon after graduating from Agricultural Chemistry Department of Chung Hsing University in Taiwan, he became our class teacher. He taught us chemistry, physics, and mathematics. He was not only young and energetic, but also dedicated and logical. Under his zeal of teaching, we began to pay attention to study. Unfortunately, in less than three years, he left us for further study in the United States. After high school, I studied at National Taiwan University Medical College. There I met many dear friends, and before I knew it, we started translating English medical literatures to Chinese and subsequently founded the *Medicine Today* journal. We did not cross path until years after I settled in New Jersey. I then met him and found out he worked with Squibb Pharmaceutical Company at New Jersey for more than thirty years and retired in 1996. His research team in the pharmaceutical company focused on the development of new anti-hypertensive medication. He was deeply involved in selecting exactly which biological pathway to suppress; designed and synthesized the potential dream compound to do the job. After years of hard work, they finally synthesized the first logical drug to suppress angiotensin-converting enzyme (ACE), i.e., Capoten or captopril, to help to control hypertension. Knowing his past discipline and talent, I am not at all surprised to learn of his groundbreaking achievement. His success did not happen by chance.

He told me after working on anti-hypertensive medication for more than thirty years he was interested to write a book about his understanding of hypertension for the general public because they have to know this very common but potentially devastating disease. I am glad he finally finished writing it. *The Mystery of Hypertension* summarizes his view on this killer. He avoids using scientific jumble mumble; instead, he uses easy, intelligible daily examples to explain hypertension. He ingeniously uses traffic jam, water in the rubber container, flow velocity of water, the pumping rate, constrictor, electric saw, office to substitute the incomprehensible medical jargons. This approach enables readers to better understand the cause and the basis of treating hypertension. The book begins with the rationale and method of measuring blood pressure, the cause of hypertension, the culprit elements that cause hypertension, and finally, the detailed listings of brand names, generic names of numerous antihypertensive drugs, including their efficacy, action mechanisms. All these are easily comprehensible because the book is written from a reader's viewpoint.

I vividly remember how he inspired us. He taught us free to postulate but be logical in drawing conclusions. One should work slowly, meticulously letting go of all the superfluous distractions and deduct carefully for the appropriate answers. Only with uncompromising determination and hard work can one achieve accurate and meaningful results. His excellent achievement is the living example of his teaching. He believes eating food after boiling them three times with water to minimize sodium and chloride intake can lower blood pressure. He used himself as a guinea pig to try this diet. He not only demonstrated its effectiveness in lowering his own blood pressures, but also revealed his discipline of self-control.

Thanks to Dr. Chi Wan Lai and Dr. Tian-Jin Chang from the editorial team of *Medicine Today* for publishing the Chinese version of this book so that he can share his view on hypertension with Chinese readers. I am most honored to have the opportunity to write the foreword in both editions—Chinese and English—for my most respected teacher who inspired us so profoundly in our early years and to recommend you an excellent book for your health.

Sun-Hoo Foo, MD, FRCP(C), FACP, FAAN
Clinical Professor of Neurology
NYU Langone Medical Center
Chief of Neurology, New York Downtown Hospital
Past Chairman, Federation of Chinese American
Chinese Canadian Medical society (FCMS)

Preface

Hypertension is a very common disease and is still listed at the top occurrence of all diseases. Even though this disease can be controlled by modern medicine, there are many patients whose blood pressure still can't be controlled enough to reach normal ranges. The reason is some factors still remain unknown.

The author tries to link these together to help the reader better understand hypertension (high blood pressure). The author also tries not to use scientific terminologies in this book and will keep the discussion at its most basic terminologies to enable the general reader to understand hypertension.

The rational drug design of Capoten® (first ACE inhibitor for the treatment of hypertension) is not intended to be discussed in this book. However, this book was published in 1998 and updated in 2003. But it is worth mentioning here that even this class of drug (ACE inhibitor) was designed for hypertension. However, recently, it has been found in a medical research from Overton Brooks VA Medical Center in Shreveport, Louisiana, that this class of drug (ACE inhibitor) was also promising only tried for three different kinds of cancers (colon, pancreas, and esophageal). Please note that this book is not to be a substitute for visiting your doctor should you have any questions or issues.

(See Web site:
http://brightsurf.com/news/headlines/24567/Blood_pressure_drugs_associated_
with_reduced_risk_of_esophageal_pancreatic_and_colon_cancers.html.)

Cheung, Hong Son

Willingboro, New Jersey
April 2008

Chapter 1

Measuring Blood Pressure

To know whether your blood pressure is high or low, you need to measure your blood pressure with conventional blood pressure measuring equipment. After such measurements, two different blood pressure values are obtained. One measurement is with a high value such as 120. The other measurement is with a low value such as 75. The high value is referred to as systolic pressure, while the low value is referred to as diastolic pressure.

The ranges between 110-120 and 68-78 are considered "normal" for systolic pressure and diastolic pressure, respectively, and has been written about and well documented in the medical arena. However, more than twenty years ago, these values had been changed to as high as 130 for systolic pressure and 90 for diastolic pressure. In recent years, it has been returned back to the above-mentioned values again. Values either below or above these ranges are considered as either hypotension (low blood pressure) or hypertension (high blood pressure), respectively. What do the systolic and diastolic pressures mean?

Even if the blood pressure values you obtain from measuring at that moment are high, this *doesn't necessarily mean you have high blood pressure and, therefore, is automatically designated as a patient with hypertension*. Judging whether the person is hypertensive or not is not just based on the high blood pressure values obtained at that moment, but must be gathered over time to determine a pattern. If the blood pressure is high at a given moment but, over a period of time, is normal most of the time, more likely than not, this person is not hypertensive.

Heart

The heart and its heartbeat contribute two (2) different major functions or steps: contraction and relaxation (Cheung 1998/2003), and two different blood pressures can be obtained simultaneously from this same single heartbeat.

A.   Contraction

The function of the contraction of the heart is to pump and push the blood out from the heart and into the artery. The pressure applied for pumping and pushing the blood from the heart into the artery during this contraction cycle is referred to as systolic pressure. Thus the systolic pressure is the power in which blood can be moved in the blood vessels during the contraction step in a heartbeat.

B.   Relaxation

The function of relaxation is the amount of blood being pumped and pushed out from the heart into the artery during the contraction cycle, and then this amount (volume) of blood returns back into the heart in the relaxation cycle. The pressure exerted to the heart by the amount of the blood returning back to fill the heart chamber in the relaxation cycle is referred to as a diastolic pressure. Thus the diastolic pressure is the power of that amount of blood residing in the heart during the relaxation step of the same heartbeat.

Blood Pressure Measuring

Four thousand years ago, the Chinese emperor Huang-Ti was already aware of the importance of the changing characteristics of pulse. With remarkable prescience of the characteristic pattern of the pulse, he concluded that people who ate too much salt had an extremely good chance of having a harder pulse movement in the wrist—which resulted from the feeling of the finger touching this position—and thus tended to suffer strokes (O'Brien and Fitzgerald 1994; Cheung 1998/2003).

However, he could only diagnose the pulse pattern but couldn't have been aware of blood pressure values due to the lack of measuring equipment available at that time.

The blood pressure monitor is well-known today and is widely used by health-care professionals and patients. It is used to measure the systemic arterial pressure through the use of a cuff with an inflatable bladder worn around the patient's arm. Then a stethoscope is used to listen to the sounds in the brachial artery. Many health-care providers know that they are listening to "Korotkoff sounds," which was introduced by a Russian doctor and scientist whose name is Nikolai Sergeevich Korotkoff one hundred years ago (Shevchenko and Tuitlik 1996; Cheung 1998/2003).

The blood pressure can be measured with the application of the following:

1. An elastic rubber cuff is worn around the arm.
2. The pressure in the cuff is increased until the blood supply to the periphery is completely stopped.
3. Then the pressure in the cuff is decreased.
4. The stethoscope is used to listen to the pressure in the artery directly below the cuff around the arm.
5. Once the pressure falls below a certain level, the first short tones can be heard; this indicates the passage of the first pulse wave along the artery below the cuff. The blood pressure monitor reading is this first tone and corresponds to the systolic pressure.
6. With further decrease in pressure in the cuff, tones are replaced by murmurs that are followed, in turn, by second tones.
7. Finally all the sounds disappear. The moment all sounds subside, according to Korotkoff, leads to the conclusion that blood is flowing freely through the arteries. The pressure in the artery at that moment slightly exceeds the pressure in the cuff, and the monitor reading corresponds at that moment to all the sounds disappearing. The last sound to be heard corresponds to the pressure reading from the monitor reading and is referred to as the diastolic pressure.

Mechanism of Blood Pressure Measurement

The blood pressure, which is generally believed to be "measured," however, is actually detection of whether the pulse is present or not (Cheung 1998/2003). The pulse detected is located in the arm artery, which is related to the same heartbeat in the cycle of contraction and relaxation of heart. Each single beat (pulse) is derived from two different cycles (steps) of contraction and relaxation. The pressure in the contraction cycle is much higher than in the relaxation cycle (Cheung 1998/2003).

In the situation of the heartbeat, however, the pulse can be heard or detected (signal picked up) mechanically because the pulse wave is formed in this single heartbeat (Cheung 1998/2003). The pulse wave occurs from the condition of heart pressures of contraction and relaxation during a one single pulse (heartbeat).

Contraction produces high pressure, and relaxation results in low pressure. In the same heartbeat (pulse), the pressures from the heart contraction and relaxation steps generate a pattern (directions) of high pressure and then low pressure, respectively.

In this single pulse (heartbeat), in the contraction step, the heart generates the high pressure, and thus, pressure direction is **high** ↑ (fig. 1, 2, and 3) or as / (fig. 1, 2, and 3); then in the relaxation step, the heart generates low pressure, and pressure direction is **low** ↓ (fig. 1, 2, and 3) or as \ (fig. 1, 2, and 3). Thus in this single heartbeat, these two different pressure directions combine together and construct the high-low pattern ↑↓ or as / \, finally closed together to the form ∧ (fig. 1) and also as a true pulse wave for this single pulse.

The pulse wave formed is the pressure direction changing or shifting from the original direction either "high to low" or "low to high" in this same single heartbeat. This direction-changing symptom, thus, can be picked up by the stethoscope or monitor with the sound mode for this single pulse (Cheung 1998/2003). The next pulse repeats the same pattern again, and sound also can be picked up or detected again and again by the monitor or stethoscope. Without the pulse wave, the changing of the pressure direction is not happening. The monitor or stethoscope, thus, cannot pick up the sound. As discussed before, whether the sound can be picked up or not is strictly dependent on whether there is a change in the direction of the pressure. Without such change, the monitor can't detect it.

In measuring the blood pressure, the pulse—heard or detected—can be measured through the use of a stethoscope and by a cuff wrapped around the arm (now also around wrist or thumb). An external pressure must be applied. In fact, the external pressure applied for that pulse must be in the range between the highest pressure and the lowest pressure of the heart itself—normal systolic and diastolic pressures, respectively

(Cheung 1998/2003). If the applied external pressure is either higher than the normal systolic or lower than diastolic pressure, no pulse can be heard or detected.

However, without the presence of measuring equipment, to detect the sound from the heart in the arm position is nearly impossible. This is due to the pulse being too weak to be detected even with the use of a stethoscope (Cheung 1998/2003).

To detect or hear the sound (pulse) around the arm, a booster (amplified) is required. The elastic, inflatable cuff must be used to wrap around the arm and, at that position, to apply external pressure with a rubber bulb connected to the cuff. This booster uses three different pressures to achieve the goal and to recreate the above-mentioned pressure pattern (directions) of the heart for same single heartbeat. After recreating the pattern to the original pressure direction, the sound can then be easily heard and detected in this fashion for each single pulse without any problems (Cheung 1998/2003).

In these three pressures, one of the pressures is external pressure applied around the arm by the elastic, inflatable cuff. The stethoscope must be in this position of the artery near the booster (amplified). The other two pressures are natural heart pressures: normal systolic pressure (highest) and normal diastolic pressure (lowest). The applied external pressure must be in the range between these two natural heart pressures to detect the heartbeat. Then the pulse (sound) can be heard and detected with the aid of a stethoscope (Cheung 1998/2003). The application of the external pressure, if higher or lower than either the systolic or diastolic pressures, will result in the sound not being picked up or detected at all by the monitor.

Beginning with increasing external pressure in the cuff around the arm to a point, the application of the external pressure must be much higher than the normal systolic pressure (natural highest heart pressure). In the contraction step, the **higher** external pressure applied is now against the **lower** natural heart pressure (in this case, it is the normal systolic pressure) for this single heartbeat. Then it generates the "pressure direction" from **high to low** ↓ or \ (fig. 1 and 2) because it is **high** external pressure against **low** systolic pressure in contraction step.

Then **in the relaxation cycle in the same heartbeat**, this external pressure is higher than systolic pressure and certainly still much higher than the normal diastolic pressure (second natural lowest heart pressure). In this condition, it still is the high external pressure against low diastolic pressure also against both low systolic and diastolic pressures simultaneously. Thus the "pressure direction" in relaxation step is also generated from **high to low** ↓ or \ (fig. 2). The combination of both "pressure directions" together from the contraction and relaxation cycles constructs the form of ↓↓ or \\ (fig. 2) for that single pulse, same heartbeat.

However, the form of pulse wave ∧ (fig. 1 and 2) certainly won't be the result for this single pulse. No pulse wave can be constructed; therefore, no change in pressure direction is certainly occurring in this pattern. Thus the blood pressure monitor can't pick up or hear the sound of such pulse (Cheung 1998/2003).

For the point to be able to detect the pulse, as mentioned above, the external pressure must be in the range between the systolic and diastolic pressures. The external pressure applied on the arm must be decreasing until, under the case, the applied external pressure is between the ranges of systolic and diastolic pressures. However, it reaches a critical point of pressure value that is **just below** the normal systolic pressure (natural highest heart pressure) in the **contraction cycle**.

Now the application of the external pressure is just **lower** than the normal systolic pressure (natural highest heart pressure). The pattern of the pressure direction in this case is **lower** applied external pressure against the **higher** natural heart systolic pressure. It is from **low to high** and then generates the form of ↑ or / (fig. 3) in the contraction cycle for this heartbeat.

Then continuing to the relaxation cycle in the same heartbeat, this external pressure begins between the ranges of the two heart pressures. The external pressure is **below** the normal systolic pressure. It is certainly **much higher** than the normal diastolic pressure (lowest natural heart pressure). Thus the pressure direction is from **higher** external pressure to the **lower** normal diastolic pressure (natural lowest heart pressure), and the pressure direction must be **high to low** ↓ or \ (fig. 1 and 2) in the relaxation cycle for same heartbeat.

Combining both pressures' direction from contraction and relaxation steps in the same heartbeat results to a pressure with the pattern ↑↓ and / \, finally constructing the pulse wave ∧ (fig. 2). The pressure direction is certainly changing. Thus the monitor can pick up and detect this sound. This is the first sound (pulse wave) detected from the blood pressure monitor (Cheung 1998/2003). This applied external pressure for the first sound detected is the value of the first blood pressure reading obtained for the systolic pressure value (Cheung 1998/2003).

The applied external pressure keeps falling but is still between the range of systolic and diastolic pressures (two natural heart pressures) for each heartbeat. The pulse waves are occurring continuously for each following heartbeat because it is still between the range of systolic and diastolic pressures. Therefore, the sound following each heartbeat can be picked up and detected by the monitor (fig. 3) until ∧ (fig. 2) is no longer present (Cheung 1998/2003).

Until the applied external pressure decreases to just below the normal diastolic pressure (lowest natural heart pressure), the external pressure is no longer between the range of the systolic and diastolic pressures (two natural heart pressures) for the heartbeat. At this moment, the applied external pressure is certainly lower than both the pressure values of the highest and lowest natural heart pressures in both cycles of contraction and relaxation in this heartbeat.

In this case, **low** external pressure is measured against both **high** systolic and diastolic pressures. Thus both the pressure directions for this pulse are **low to high** and designated as ↑↑ or // (fig. 2). Therefore, ∧ (fig. 1) is no longer present. Because both pressure directions found are the same without changing, sound (pulse wave) can no longer be detected and picked up (Cheung 1998/2003). For the following heartbeat, the external pressure is no longer between the ranges of the two natural heart pressures (systolic and diastolic), and it would be lower than both natural heart pressures. As a result, the pulse wave won't be found anymore, and the direction of the changing pressure no longer exists. The sound of the following heartbeats won't be heard and detected by the monitor again.

However, the last sound detected is from the case of the application of the external pressure just **above** the normal diastolic pressure (lowest heart natural pressure). It is a **high** external pressure against a **low** diastolic pressure. The pressure direction is **high to low** designated as ↓ or \ for the relaxation step in the heartbeat. However, the last sound detected is under the condition that the external pressure is applied between the pressures of the systolic and diastolic pressures. Naturally, this external pressure is still **lower** than the **high** systolic pressure. Therefore, the pressure pattern is ↑ or / for the contraction step in the same heartbeat. Thus the direction of both pressure patterns combined are ↑↓ and / \ and is finally designated as the pulse wave ∧. This is the last wave, which could be formed for that pulse. This is the last detected sound (pulse wave) of applied external pressure from the monitor, and its value is the blood pressure reading collected and defined as the diastolic pressure (Cheung 1998/2003).

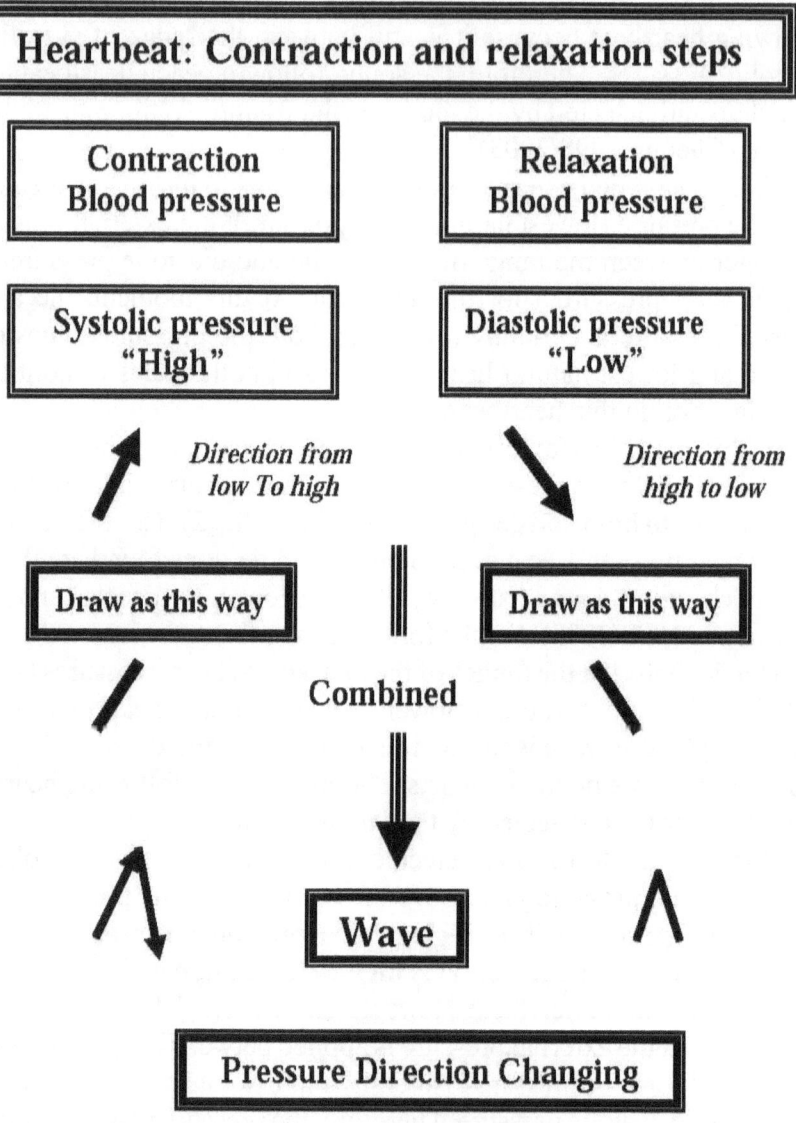

Fig. 1. Mechanism of Blood Pressure Measurement
By The Monitor (A)

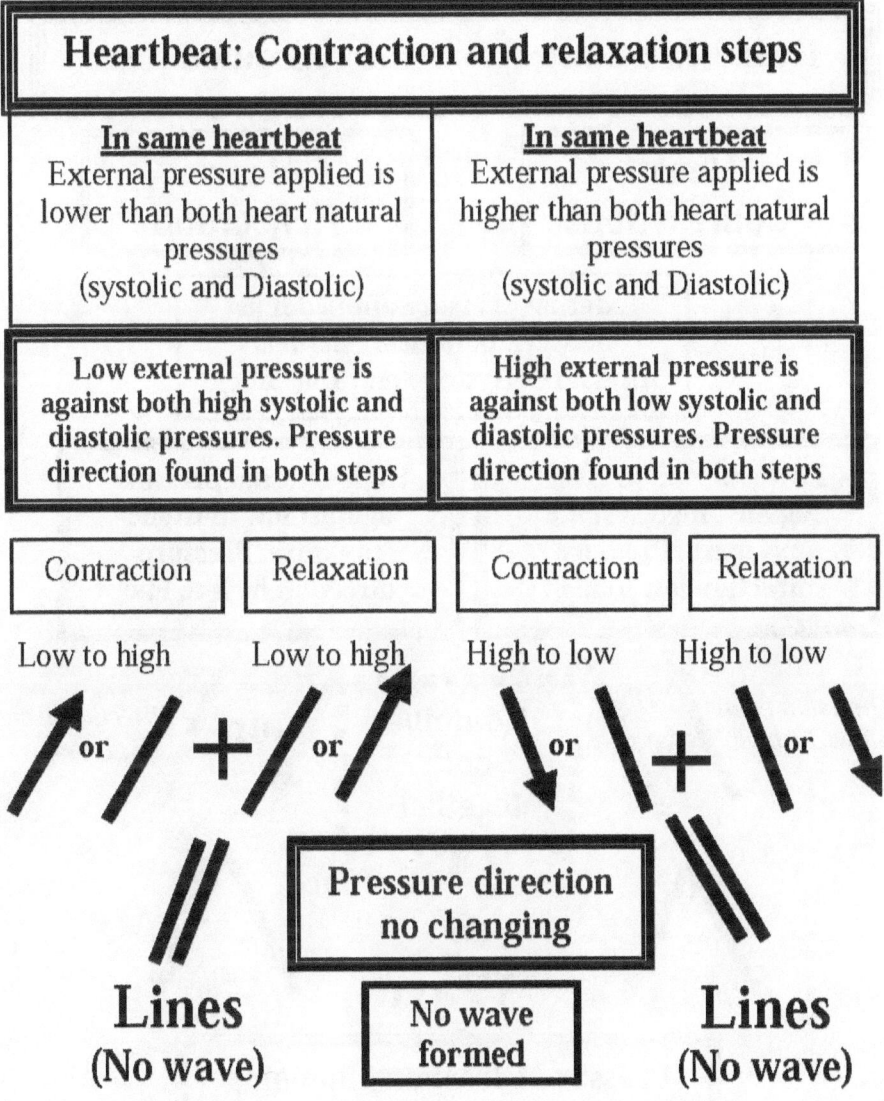

Fig. 2. Mechanism of Blood Pressure Measurement
By The Monitor (B)

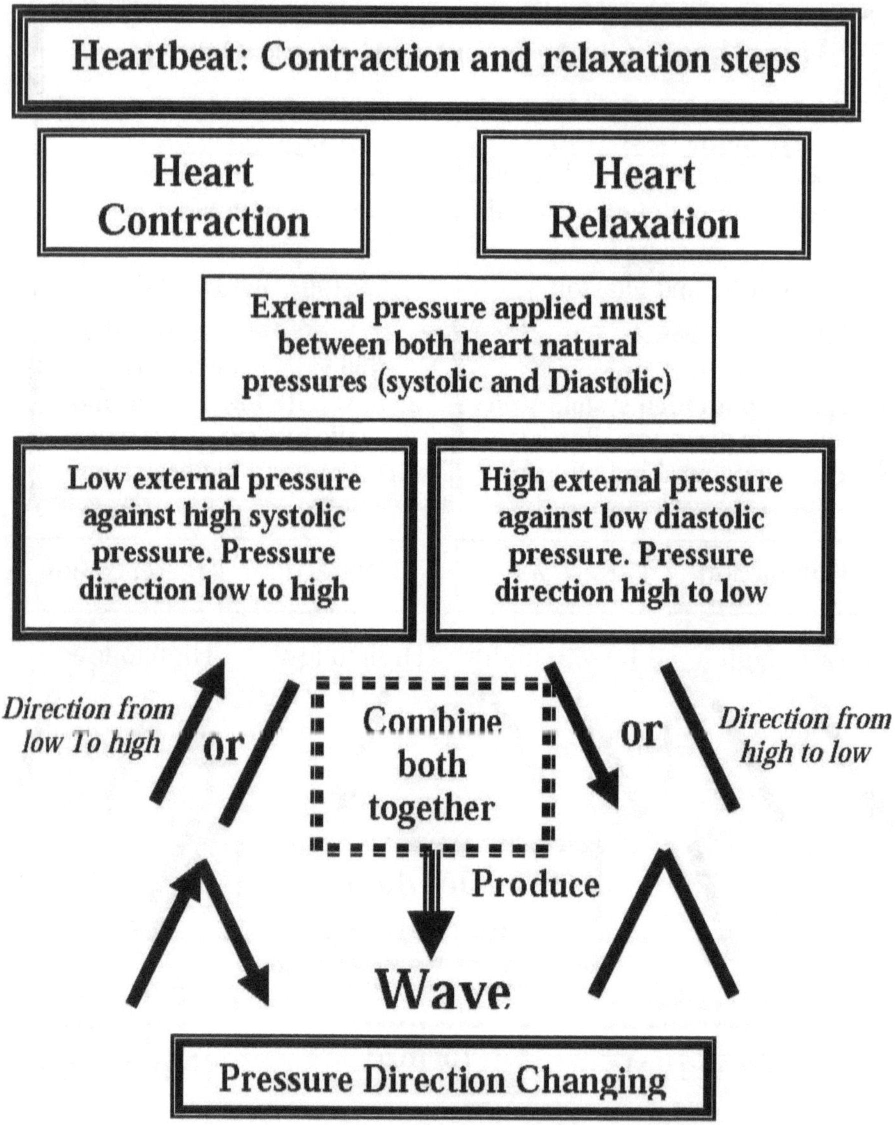

Heartbeat: Contraction and relaxation steps

Heart Contraction

Heart Relaxation

External pressure applied must between both heart natural pressures (systolic and Diastolic)

Low external pressure against high systolic pressure. Pressure direction low to high

High external pressure against low diastolic pressure. Pressure direction high to low

Direction from low To high

or

Combine both together

or

Direction from high to low

Produce

Wave

Pressure Direction Changing

Fig. 3. Mechanism of Blood Pressure Measurement
By The Monitor (C)

Even both values of systolic and diastolic pressures are obtained from the monitor. However, they are not true systolic and diastolic pressure values for heart. As discussed above, both of these values of systolic and diastolic pressures, which are collected from the monitor, are just below and above the true systolic and diastolic pressures, respectively. Therefore, those collected heart pressures values are just a little lower or higher than the true heart (systolic and diastolic) pressure values, respectively. However, the difference found in the blood pressures between the collected and the true values of heart are so little even they are different, but they are insignificant. Thus the collected values are still meaningful.

During blood pressure measuring, some found that the blood pressures obtained after remeasuring one or two times are usually lower than the first measured values. The question is which one should be considered as the correct one?

Usually, before the measuring, we already performed some activity such as walking. This activity will raise your heart rate a little faster and thus resulting to the blood pressure also being raised a little higher. Before you measure your pressure, you should sit a while to allow your heart rate to **return back to normal**, and hence blood pressure drops back to normal. Therefore, in this case, remeasuring the value is more meaningful.

Chapter 2

Pressure Occurring in Related Natural Condition

To understand blood pressure, we must first be aware of the related natural pressure. In the following section, we try to discuss it.

The heart functions, not unlike the example of a rubber container, to hold the blood in the circulatory system of the human body. This heart (rubber container) also serves as a powerful pump to pump and to push the blood out to the artery and vessels. Then the blood is circulated and passed throughout the body. If this circulating system is functioning normally, the blood flowing in the artery and vessels are also normal. The blood pressure in this environment (circulating system) is generally normal.

The three cases are as follows:

A. The flow rate of the blood in the system is decreasing.
B. The amount of blood in the heart is more than it is supposed to be.
C. The heartbeat is increased.

In the occurrence of any such cases, which deviates from the normal, the function of the heart can change from normal to abnormal. Usually, the resulting blood pressure can be higher than normal in such situations. This is the simplest explanation to describe why hypertension has occurred.

The three scenarios above are discussed as follows:

A. Flow rate of the blood in the system is decreasing.

       The flow rate of the blood under the normal or perfect condition is when the blood can move and flow freely in the artery and vessels. However, in the case, where there is resistance or some interruption during the flow of blood in the system, the flow rate will be decreased. Thus the lowering of the flow rate may result in a higher blood pressure than normal.

B. The amount of blood in the heart (container) is more than it is supposed to be.

An increase in the amount of blood in the heart can cause the container to be at overcapacity. Thus the heart will feel heavier and have to work harder, which could result to an increase in the blood pressure in heart.

C. The rate of heartbeat is increased.

Mechanically, after the pumping in the system, a pressure will result. The pressure, either high or low, will be directly proportional to the pumping rate of the system. Thus, a faster pumping rate will result in a higher pressure, and vice versa. Otherwise, a lower pumping rate will result to a lower pressure.

From the above explanations, these three factors can cause the blood pressure to rise. However, the most important factors are the first two: flow rate of the blood in the circulating system and increased amounts of blood in the heart. These two factors can play major roles in causing hypertension.

Here are examples from related natural pressure.

A. Flow rate of the *water* in the circulating system.

Water can be used as a substitute for blood, and a water hose can replace the blood vessels. Water would be flowing in the water hose.

a. As mentioned above, there is a resistance or interruption occurring during the flow in the system. As a result, the pressure will most likely rise. What can cause the resistance or interruption? Why does the resistance affect the pressure in the circulating system?

To answer these questions, consider the following examples.

Water flows in the water hose, and there is a water pressure in the hose. The water pressure, high or low, strictly depends on the amount of water flowing through it. If a constant amount of water flows through the hose, the water pressure in the hose will also remain constant.

In the case where the hose has been used for many years—in nature, due to deterioration—the hose wall will probably become harder than normal. The water pressure found in this hard hose will rise even if it is the same amount of water running through this hose.

For example, if anyone has ever tried to partially cover the hose opening with his/her hands or fingers (decreasing the hose opening size, diameter), the water pressure in this partially covered hose is increased automatically, and the flow rate of the water prior to the opening is also found to slow down.

Thus it also can be summarized as follows:

1. Naturally, the hose, which becomes harder, increases the water pressure when compared to the hose when new or not too old.
2. This increased water pressure is also observed from the smaller diameter (size of opening) of the water hose by partially covering the opening (as demonstrated above).

By partially covering the hose's opening, the water flow in the hose prior to the opening is decreased. A higher water pressure is also found from this resistance (blocking) occurring in the partially covered area of the hose. Thus it is not just the decrease of the diameter of the hose affecting the resistance, but also any resistance or blockage of the hose affecting the water flow. Thus a decreased opening size (diameter) of the hose thereby has higher resistance and higher water pressure, and vice versa (increased opening size of hose, low resistance and low water pressure could occur).

As a result, a higher water pressure can be found from both occurrence of an older hose hardened by nature and a hose with a small-diameter opening (size) from example above. Certainly, the harder hose having higher water pressure must have the same reason as the hose with smaller-diameter opening (size).

Therefore, it can be concluded as follows:

1. An older (harder) hose thereby has a higher resistance and water pressure.
2. Thus such a hose in number 1 and a small-diameter hose from the example above would result in a higher water pressure in the hose.
3. An older (harder) hose, having higher water pressure, thus, must contribute a similar reason as the smaller size of the diameter of the hose.
4. It also means that the hose after the opening size is changed to smaller would become harder. (This will be explained more fully later.)

b. Also the resistance can be increased with the occurrence of foreign material flowing into the hose. This material accumulates and then binds with the hose. As a result, there will only be a partial opening of the pathway for the movement of fluid. The diameter (size) at this blocked location in the hose is smaller. The smaller diameter found in this case will also affect the resistance. Thus the pressure should be increased also. This situation is not exactly identical with the situation as mentioned above, but the occurrences are from the same reason but without the harder hose situation happening.

B. The amount of *water* in the container is more.

The container here is used to hold water for storage. A certain fixed amount of water in the container will result in a fixed weight applied to the container. This fixed weight from a fixed amount of water will exert a pressure to the wall of the container. Therefore, there is water pressure applied to the container.

In the event that an additional amount of water is added to the container, the weight of water in the container is increased. The pressure applied to the container is also increased.

C. The pumping rate of the *container* is increased.

This container also serves as a powerful pumping machine. The process of pumping necessitates the creation of a pressure. For example, a tire and bike pump, if pumped by hand, simulates a pumping situation. You will notice and feel that there is a resulting pressure in the tire. If there is no pumping, there is no pressure observed built up in the tire. It will also be noticed that during the pumping, if the pumping is faster, the pressure found will be higher from the tire or bike pump. However, the slower the pumping, the pressure will also be low. Thus the pumping process in the rubber container also creates a pressure analogous to the tire pump.

For this reason, a fast rate of pumping certainly produces higher pressure, and a lower rate produces lower pressure. Thus the pumping rate is also a factor, which can result to hypertension.

Chapter 3

Blood Pressure Occurring in the Heart

We discussed blood pressure in chapter 1.

In chapter 2, three (3) different cases/analogies were mentioned, which could affect the blood pressure:

A. The flow rate of the water in the system is decreased.
B. The amount of water in the container is increased beyond normal.
C. The pumping rate of the container is increased.

This will result in the behavior of the water changing from normal to abnormal. Usually, the water pressure will be found to be higher than normal in such circumstances.

In chapter 2, we discussed pressures with the example of water. We will now compare this with the blood pressure in the heart.

A. **The flow rate of the *blood* in the system is slowed down.**

In the following examples, the heart replaces the container and blood replaces the water in the system. Combining them together becomes a blood and heart circulating system. During the contraction cycle, blood is being pumped out from the heart and then enters into the artery and vessels and then circulates in the blood vessels. The blood pressure found in this situation is referred to as **systolic pressure**. In the event that the blood vessels are constricted by some reasons, a smaller diameter of blood vessels can occur. After blood vessels are constricted, the vessels can also become tighter. The tightening process will result to a harder vessel. Therefore, as discussed in chapter 2 using the example of water, the smaller the diameter of the **hose**, the lower the flow rate and the harder the hose. And a higher water pressure will be observed. With respect to the blood and heart, after the blood vessels constrict, the size (diameter) of the vessels would be decreased. From the explanation in chapter 2, the hard water hose contributing the higher water pressure is from the smaller diameter of the opening of the hose. Therefore, for this same reason, the vessels constricted with a smaller size of opening will certainly also become harder. The blood pressure in this situation in the vessels definitely will be found to be higher.

Thus it can be concluded here that when the blood vessels are constricted, the results are as follows:

1. The diameter of blood vessels is decreased.
2. Blood vessels become harder.

As a result, the flow rate of blood is certain to slow down, leading to an increase in blood pressure.

B.   The amount of *blood* in the heart is more.

A certain normal amount of blood is held in the heart. This amount (volume) of blood and its related weight will exert a certain pressure to the walls of heart. This kind of blood pressure is referred to as **diastolic pressure**.

It also can be demonstrated by using air and a balloon. When blowing air into the balloon, we can feel that there is a pressure in the balloon. The pressure—whether high or low—is strictly dependent on how much air has been blown into the balloon. The more air in the balloon, the more the pressure will increase in the balloon, and conversely, the less air in the balloon, the lower the pressure will be found.

The balloon can also be looked at as the heart, and the air is represented as blood. Thus, for the same reason, the blood in the heart will contribute to a pressure exerted on the heart. This blood pressure is referred to as **diastolic pressure**. Thus the more blood in the heart, the higher the blood pressure (diastolic pressure) is. And when it contracts, the less blood in the heart, the lower the blood pressure (diastolic pressure) should be.

This pressure, which is natural, will always and be automatically present, and the amount of blood in the heart certainly will contribute that much pressure naturally occurring in the heart. This is the smallest blood pressure—a basic pressure also acting as a control pressure in the heart. **This defined diastolic pressure is completely different from all others.**

C.   The rate of *heartbeat* is increased.

As mentioned in chapter 2, pumping creates a pressure. Therefore, a heartbeat (heart pumping) also creates blood pressure. A higher heartbeat (pumping) rate results in higher blood pressure, and a lower heartbeat rate is found to have a lower blood pressure.

The increased rate of heartbeat can occur from activities such as exercising, doing heavy lifting, being anxious or worried, etc. Most likely, the blood pressure is raised. However, after such activities/events have stopped, the rate of the heartbeat will be gradually returned back to normal, and the blood pressure will be lowered back to normal. This kind of pressure that arises is normal and fine and is not considered as hypertension. Unless, of course, the rate of the heartbeat remains high and does not return back to normal. Then the blood pressure will stay high too. In this case, it will be considered as hypertension. This can usually be treated by the medication β-blocker to lower the heartbeat rate and the higher blood pressure.

Chapter 4

Categories of Hypertension

In this chapter, the categories of hypertension will be discussed.

Usually, there are two major kinds of hypertension. They are the following:

1. Vasoconstriction (constriction)
2. Water retention

There is another kind of symptom that can also cause hypertension and can occur from a large amount of cholesterol found in the system, which may accumulate on the walls of the artery or vessel and, thus, partially blocking the flowing pathway. It thus decreases the flow of blood because the pathway is blocked. The opening size of the vessels is smaller. Therefore, the blood pressure would also be found to be higher in this case (refer to the case A-b in chapter 2). In more serious cases, as the pathways are blocked more, the circulating blood could be completely stopped or the flow of blood could be very slow. This can lead to a heart attack or stroke. Generally, this case is considered as the natural cause of a heart attack or stroke and certainly is related to hypertension.

1. Vasoconstriction (Constriction)

This is also referred to as case A in chapters 2 and 3.

If the vessel is constricted (vasoconstriction) in the human body, after constriction, the blood vessels will be harder, and its diameter is smaller. The resistance in the vessels will increase.

Why and how can the vessels be constricted inside the human body?

To answer this question, a hypertensive agent (vasoconstrictor or constrictor) is produced inside our body (Skeggs et al. 1954/1956; Cheung 1998/2003; Cushman and Cheung 1971/1972). In biochemical terms, a hypertensive agent (vasoconstrictor) is called angiotensin II (Skeggs et al. 1954/1956; Cheung 1998/2003; Cushman and Cheung 1971/1972), which is a substance having the powerful ability to constrict the blood vessels and, thus, leading to the results of hypertension.

How can a hypertensive agent be produced inside the human body?

For example, the making of a product on the market used in our daily life, such as a desk, are all made in some way by a machine. A desk requires a machine to make it. To cut the wood, an electric saw, which is a machine, is required. In other words, for a product to be made, a machine is required for this task.

For the purpose of producing or making anything, such as the hypertensive agent, vasoconstrictor or angiotensin II (Skeggs et al. 1954/1956; Cheung 1998/2003; Cushman and Cheung 1971/1972), in the human body, the human machine is also required to perform this job. This human machine "enzymes" within the body manufacture a constrictor (angiotensin II, hypertensive agent) called angiotensin-converting enzyme (ACE) (Skeggs et al. 1954/1956; Cheung 1998/2003; Cushman and Cheung 1971/1972). The angiotensin-converting enzyme is one of the specific enzymes (machines) in the human body.

From now on in this book, for definition purposes, the name of **constrictor will be used to replace the name of angiotensin II, hypertensive agent, or vasoconstrictor. The machine will represent an enzyme.** Again, in the following example, **the machine is used to make the constrictor inside of the human body. The constrictor constricts the blood vessels, thereby resulting to harder vessels and decreased diameter of vessels. This symptom will most likely result to a higher blood pressure.**

There are many, many different machines in the human body tasked to do different jobs to make different human products. The specific constrictor machine (angiotensin-converting enzyme) is the one machine that plays the role of manufacturing the "constrictor" in the human body. The constrictor machine will be mentioned as a machine later in this book.

After the constrictor is made by the machine, it will travel around the body, and then arriving at its office, it stays there (binding) and works there. This office is also named as a "receptor" (Chiu et al. 1988/1990; Wong et al. 1989), a specific term in biochemistry, and will be referred to as "office" hereinafter.

This office is just like a power station. The operator works in the power station and operates the equipment, which then delivers the electric power to each house to light their lamps and also to their appliances.

The constrictor arrives to its office to do its work just as the operator in the power station situation. Then the constrictor (operator) in his office can control and operate the equipment to do his work of constricting blood vessels for the entire body.

The blood vessel, after it is constricted, becomes tighter and much close together then and becomes a harder vessel, and the diameter of the vessel is also smaller. With the smaller opening size of vessels and harder vessels, from the facts and explanation in chapter 3, the flowing rate of the blood should be found to decrease; and also because of the smaller opening size of vessels and harder vessels, the blood pressure is higher.

The increased amount of constrictors produced in the body arrives and occupies more offices in our body simultaneously. More offices will work together to constrict the vessels. The ability to constrict the vessels should be much more powerful. Thus vessels, after this constricted condition, will become much harder, and the diameter of the vessel will be much smaller. A more increased blood pressure would be found under this condition (fig. 4). However, in this case, when a decreased amount of constrictors are produced, fewer number of offices will be occupied by the constrictors. Certainly, the ability to constrict the blood vessels will be much less. The vessel will be less constricted, and the blood pressure will be found to be lower (fig. 4).

Thus higher systolic pressure is certainly the result of increased amounts of constrictors being produced in the body, then leading to the smaller size of the vessel (harder vessel) and slowing down of the flow rate also occurring in the body.

2.   Water Retention

This is referred to as case B in chapters 2 and 3.

A long time ago, it was recognized that high blood pressure resulted from water retention (Cheung 2003). Water retention means more amounts of water are held inside the human body leading to an excess beyond the normal amount. Table salt (sodium chloride) has been known to cause water retention by Western and Chinese physicians for a long time (fig. 5) (Cheung 2003).

More water in the human body could result in high blood pressure. This general opinion is even widely agreed upon by the medical society. However, even though its acceptance is already known in general, is it clear how and why the rise in blood pressure only occurs in the vessels and the heart but not observed anywhere in the body?

The blood pressure, being higher, is clearly and strictly related to the vessels and hearts. Thus the above accepted point of **more water in the human body** will result to the higher blood pressure certainly is not entirely accurate. Rather it should be more appropriately changed to say **more water** in the *heart and vessels* and not the body (fig. 6).

After clarifying and indicating that blood pressure is related to the *heart and vessels*, it can be used easily to explain the following.

Blood is a very complicated substance and contains many soluble and insoluble materials in suspension. However, the major component of the blood is water. Thus the more water in the blood, the more the volume of blood will be increased. Due to more water in the heart, the total amount (volume) of blood is increased in the heart. The more blood in the heart, the blood pressure is, of course, increased (explanation in chapter 3). In this case, the higher blood pressure here is referred to the raised diastolic pressure.

Therefore, the higher diastolic pressure should be a result from more blood in the heart.

Thus it can be concluded as follows:

1. Constriction results in a higher systolic pressure in a contraction step in a heartbeat.
2. Water retention results in a higher diastolic pressure in a relaxation step in the same heartbeat.

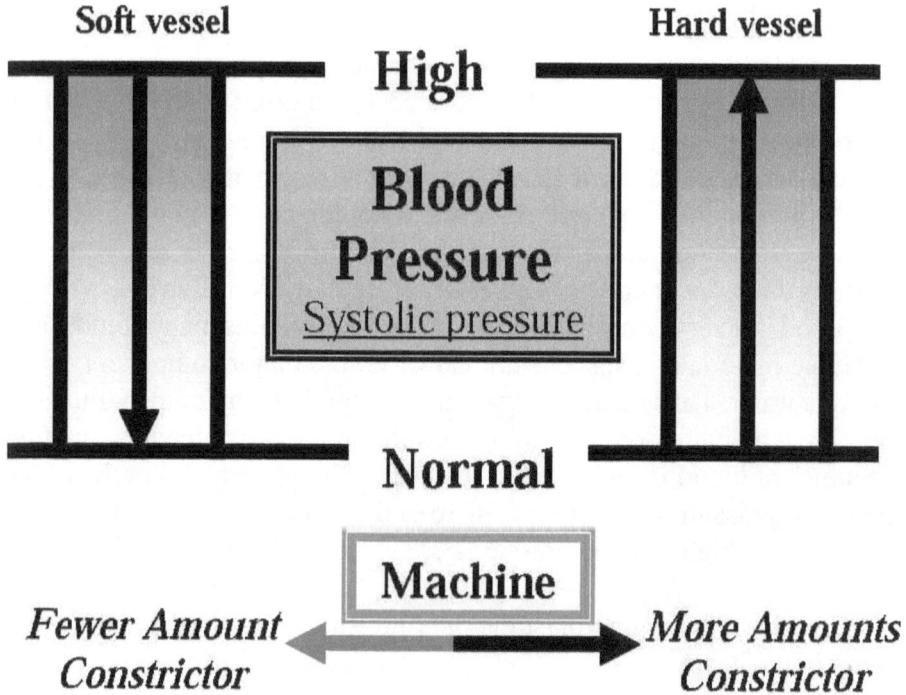

Fig. 4. Relationship of Blood Pressure
and The Amount of Constrictor

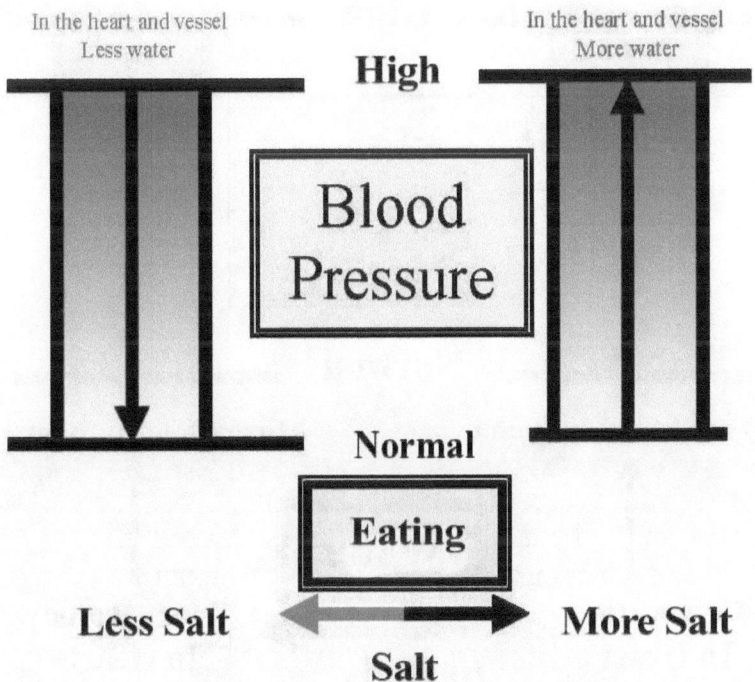

Fig. 5. Relationship of Blood Pressure
and The Amount of Sodium Chloride

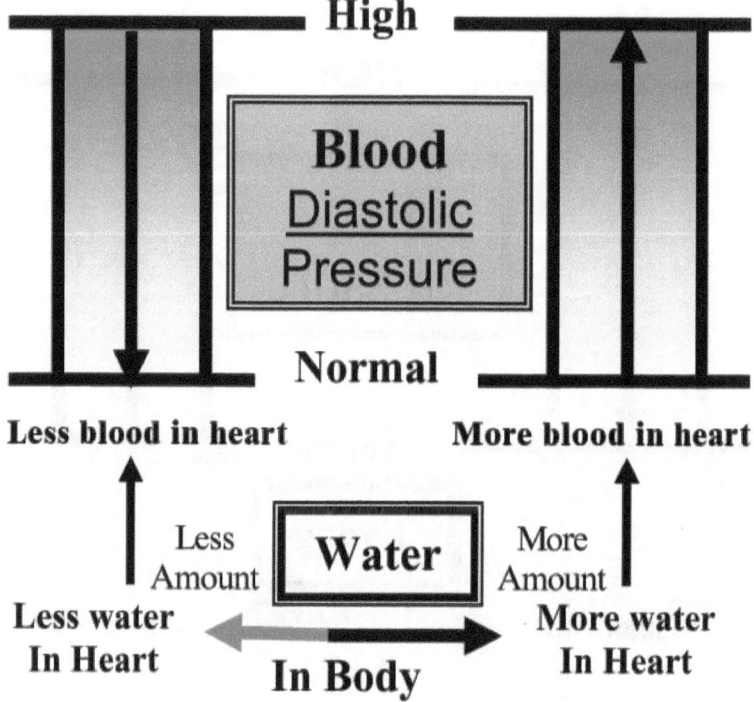

Fig. 6. Relationship of Blood Pressure
and Blood Volume (Amount) in the Heart

Chapter 5

Diet Causes Hypertension

In this chapter, we are going to discuss the relationship between diet and hypertension.

We have discussed the blood pressure and function and its relation to increased blood pressure. However, what external factors can cause hypertension? As discussed before, we understand the mechanism of hypertension, and now, we discuss causes from this external factor.

It is commonly known that some substances such as salt will cause an increase in blood pressure. However, what is the true substance that can cause an increase in blood pressure?

As mentioned in previous chapters, there are only two different blood pressures found in the heart. One is high blood pressure value (systolic pressure). The other is low value (diastolic pressure). Either one or both values of systolic or diastolic pressure higher will be considered as hypertension. These two different blood pressures occur from two different functions of the heart, the steps of contraction and relaxation, in the same heartbeat. Therefore, only these two blood pressures would be concerned for hypertension.

So the question to be answered is which substance simultaneously causes both functions of hypertension in the body, both systolic and diastolic pressures higher, and which substance possibly does this?

As discussed above, salt is known to cause hypertension. It must be clarified that there are many different kind of salts such as sodium salt (including table salt, Accent [sodium glutamate], and so on), potassium salt, and others.

All salt, including sodium salt (not including table salt), may cause some forms of hypertension. However, salt by itself is not the real and true factor resulting in hypertension. Some salts don't even cause high blood pressure. *The salt, the real and true one, is table salt.* Only table salt will trigger both functions of constriction (vasoconstriction) and water retention in hypertension simultaneously. Other salts only trigger one of the two functions or may not trigger any at all. This is the reason why table salt is the true enemy for hypertension.

To be qualified and defined as a real and true agent (enemy) for causing hypertension, this substance must trigger both the functions of constriction and water retention simultaneously in vessels and heart. In other words, both systolic and diastolic blood pressures will be high. Why is it table salt?

Table salt is also known as sodium chloride in chemistry and will be referred to as such hereinafter.

To qualify as a real and true agent for causing blood pressure to increase higher, it must trigger and cause both the systolic and diastolic pressure to be raised. This external substance must be introduced from eating frequently and taking in an amount too much.

If the substance triggers only one of the functions, one of the blood pressures can be increased. This substance should not be considered as a real cause for high blood pressure. The reason one of the blood pressures found even higher is from this substance. However, after this substance is removed from the body, certainly this blood pressure returns to normal. In fact, the other blood pressure could still remain high. You still have high blood pressure. For this reason, this substance should not be considered as a real and true agent for causing hypertension.

Why does sodium chloride control both functions? Other salts don't.

As mentioned above, systolic blood pressure is the result of constriction (vasoconstriction). Diastolic blood pressure is from water retention.

Constriction occurs from more constrictors (hypertension agents) produced in the human body. The presence of more constrictors will constrict the blood vessels even more and certainly raises the systolic pressure even higher. This is related to the function of the contraction step in the heartbeat.

However, the other function of the heartbeat is the relaxation step. Water retention occurs from too much water held in the heart as explained in chapters 3 and 4. Thus the diastolic blood pressure is high because of water retention. This higher diastolic pressure is related to the function in the relaxation step of the heartbeat.

Sodium chloride is contributing to both of these functions in nature.

Sodium chloride is a substance, a table salt, and a chemical compound. In the old days, fresh table salt was purchased from the market and stored in the bowl in the kitchen and would be used for cooking. After many days later, water would gradually be present in the bowl on top of the salt. Why does this occur in the bowl with the stored sodium chloride and is not present in a bowl without sodium chloride? Because sodium chloride has a strong ability to absorb water (moisture) from the air. This is the reason why water will be present in the bowl on the top of the salt.

This is also the reason why medical professionals always warn their patients to take lesser amounts of table salt (sodium chloride) in order to lower their blood pressure, thereby removing more water from the body. Because without sodium chloride present, the function of water absorption will also disappear. And thus the presence of water in the body will also be decreased. The high blood pressure, therefore, would also be decreased. This situation is just identical with the finding from above that table salt absorbed the water in the bowl. And no doubt, table salt has a strong ability to absorb water into the human body.

In chapter 4, it has been explained that the more water absorbed in the body, the more water would be found present in the body. It also induces more water into the heart. The major component of blood is water. More water in the heart will certainly increase the blood volume. Thus more blood will also result in the heart. As a result of explanation above, the absorption of water by sodium chloride will cause more total volume of blood in the heart. And the blood pressure will also be higher, as discussed before, from the increased total volume of blood in the heart. Thus sodium chloride causing hypertension certainly is related to the function of water retention. The heart's diastolic pressure, thus, is also found to be higher in this situation. This is also in the relaxation step of the heartbeat.

Thus this explains how sodium chloride controls the function for hypertension in the heart. However, it is just for water retention, the diastolic pressure in the relaxation step of the heartbeat.

But how can sodium chloride also relate to the other function, the contraction step in the same heartbeat, and the higher or lower systolic pressure?

As explained in chemistry, a property of sodium chloride is its strong ability to absorb water. This property will trigger a higher blood pressure.

To go deeper, the property to absorb water is not from sodium chloride itself but rather is from the sodium (sodium ion) alone. It is because of the presence of sodium in sodium chloride, which has this strong ability to absorb water. With this clarification, any sodium salt such as Accent (sodium glutamate) should have this same ability to absorb water. Thus sodium is the one factor affecting the function of water retention and causing higher diastolic pressure. Therefore, the higher diastolic pressure is not a result of the entire compound of sodium chloride.

Is there any possibility of another function such as constricting vessels in hypertension that is also related to sodium chloride?

The sodium chloride is a chemical compound combined from both sodium and chloride. The function of sodium in the sodium chloride substance is already explained and understood to absorb water. But is there any possibility that sodium chloride can also play the role of constricting vessels in hypertension or the part of chloride in table salt (sodium chloride) playing the role in hypertension (high blood pressure) in the human body? (Cheung 2003).

Does the chloride in sodium chloride play a role in hypertension? How important is it?

Chloride (chloride ion) does play a role in hypertension. Chloride plays an indirect role to promote the ability of the machine to produce an increased presence of constrictors (Cushman and Cheung 1972; Cheung 2003). The increased amount of the constrictors will result in the constriction of blood vessels, becoming much harder and tighter, and the opening size (diameter) of vessels becoming much smaller in diameter. With a decreased opening size, as discussed in chapters 3 and 4, the blood pressure will increase. Thus chloride does play a role indirectly in increasing or decreasing the blood pressure, and in this case, the systolic pressure. Thus chloride indirectly controls the other related function, the constriction in the contraction step in the same heartbeat.

In the same heartbeat, as mentioned in above paragraph, chloride certainly found will be to indirectly influence the function of the systolic pressure in the contraction step. However, sodium affects the other function of the same heartbeat by absorbing more water in the relaxation step in the same heartbeat to raise the diastolic pressure. Thus the presence of sodium chloride is similar with the situation of sodium and chloride presence together. Therefore, both heart functions are from the same heartbeat, and the contraction and relaxation steps would be affected with the presence of sodium chloride salt (sodium and chloride together). Naturally, both systolic and diastolic pressures are also increased with more sodium chloride presence. This is the reason why sodium chloride could control both heart functions—systolic and diastolic pressures—in same heartbeat simultaneously and, in theory, the contraction and relaxation steps.

Any other salt containing either sodium or chloride is not a sodium chloride salt. Therefore, only one of the responsible heart functions in same heartbeat could be found to occur.

Thus the following can be concluded here (fig. 7):

1. Sodium (sodium ion) controls the function of water retention (diastolic pressure) in the relaxation step in the same heartbeat.
2. Chloride (chloride ion) controls the constriction (vasoconstriction) of the vessels (systolic pressure) in contraction step in the same heartbeat.
3. Thus a single substance of sodium chloride (table salt) will control both functions of water retention and constriction in the human body. It will also control the blood pressures (systolic pressure and diastolic pressure) and both contraction and relaxation steps of the same heartbeat.

Hypertension is a kind of disease. Diseases usually require treatment through the use of drugs. However, drugs are generally designed for the treatment of a specific disease and, generally, for a specific function. Usually, the disease is certainly derived from the occurrence of one function. Therefore, drugs can be very effective for the disease in this situation. However, some diseases are derived from two or more different functions occurring together. In this case, a one-function drug, therefore, is not quite effective in controlling this kind of disease.

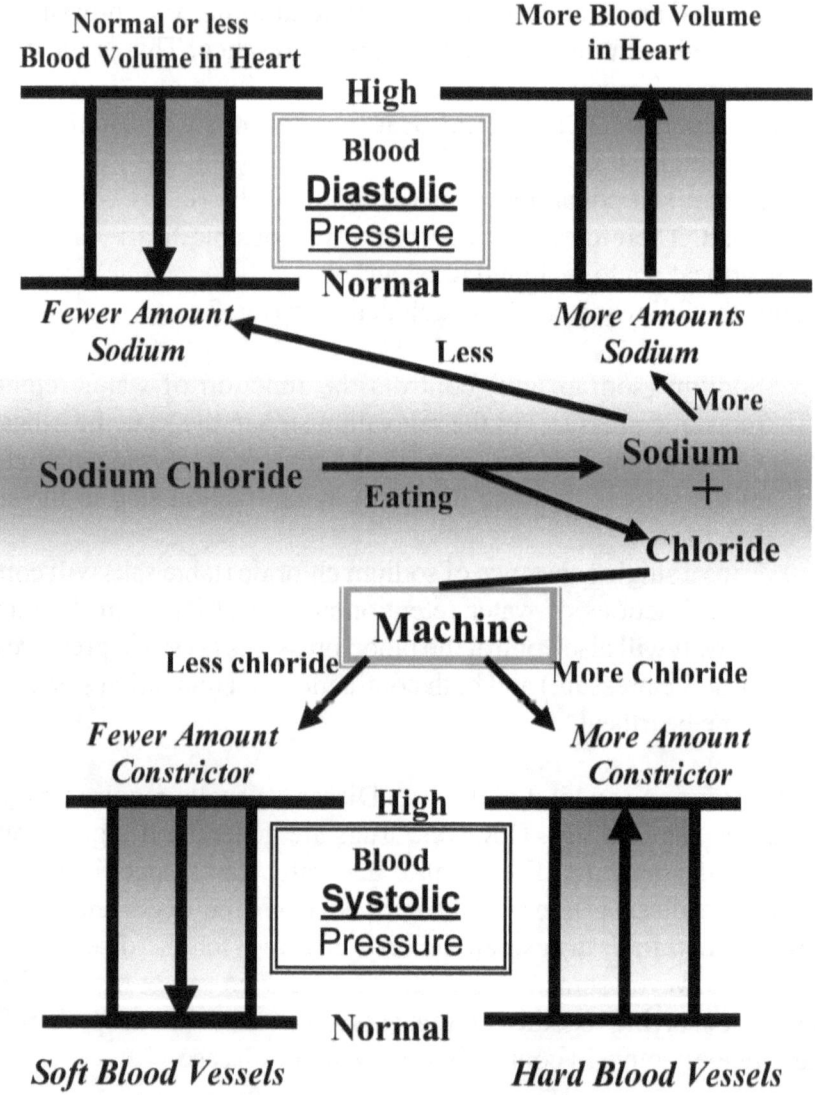

Fig. 7. Relationship of Both Diastolic and Systolic Pressures, and The Sodium Chloride (Table Salt)

Hypertension usually occurs from the combination of two different functions working together—water retention and constriction. Thus for this kind of hypertension, the one-function drug is no longer as effective and can't be expected to control the hypertension well. From this explanation, it can be readily understood why certain types of hypertension or diseases cannot be controlled by drugs in some patients. However, **if the hypertension is only from the occurrence of one function and only one of the blood pressures is higher, either systolic or diastolic pressure, the use of appropriate drugs can effectively lower the patient's blood pressure.**

Now, back to the subject of sodium chloride, and according to the concept just mentioned above, hypertension is derived from two different functions occurring together. These two functions—constriction and water retention—are the results of sodium chloride. At this moment, there is **no known single drug that can effectively control both of the functions and both the blood pressures simultaneously** unless a combination of drugs is used, one for each function in the treatment. This kind of treatment is called a **cocktail therapy**.

In some patients, the blood pressure is effectively controlled by the cocktail treatment. But in some cases, some are even effectively controlled by cocktail treatment, but with slightly different minor problems occurring because their blood pressure is lowered only to the range of 130 or higher for systolic pressure and 90 or higher for diastolic pressure. Those values cannot be further decreased by any kind of known treatment.

As discussed above, sodium chloride is the real agent causing hypertension. People eat sodium chloride every day and can consume vast quantities as measured over many years. Because of this longer length of time, the sodium chloride will accumulate in the vessel and heart wall tightly and can't be removed easily by our daily activity or drug treatment in our life. Under this condition, it would result in the blood pressure dropping with drug treatment to only about 130/90 or above, and the blood pressure can't be further dropped to the normal range as expected by any medication treatment.

To help understand why sodium chloride binds tightly and can't be easily removed from the heart and blood vessels, the following example is used. Many people enjoy drinking many cups of coffee or tea on a given day. After drinking, if you wash the cup immediately, it is very easy to clean the cup. However, some procrastinators are not going to wash the cup soon.

Some may drink little or a portion of the coffee, and a lot of it still remains in the cup. That remaining coffee usually sits in the cup for long periods of time. You will notice that these cups, after being washed, are very hard to clean and can leave a dark coffee or tea stain. Analogously, excessive amounts of sodium chloride can "stain" the vessels in the circulatory system, which can also be hard to remove and clean too.

In the heart, the sodium chloride stain cannot be removed naturally. However, simultaneous with continuously taking sodium chloride and with drug treatment, the sodium in sodium chloride will result to absorption of certain amounts of water into the heart. That amount of water volume absorbed from sodium (sodium chloride stain) will increase the total blood volume in the heart. This little increased amount of blood volume is the reason why blood pressures under drug treatment can't be lowered to 90 limiting values for diastolic pressure.

However, the other part, chloride (sodium chloride stain), would promote the production of the little more amount of constrictor in the body. This little increased amount of constrictors would also constrict blood vessels, making them harder, and would lead to a little higher blood pressure. This is also the reason why systolic pressure under drug treatment also can't be dropped lower than the 130 values.

In fact, there is a way to lower this kind of high blood pressure further. It will be discussed later in this chapter in the personal evidence section.

The role of how chloride constricts the vessels has been described. Nevertheless, I have not been able to find such clinical evidence that proves the role of chloride. The only evidence that can be found is not from the clinical studies, but from the experimentation in test-tube studies.

The ability of chloride to produce more constrictors in the test tube was the subject of experiments by the author (Cushman and Cheung 1972; Cheung 2003). If there is a chloride found in the human body, why could this chloride not have the ability to decide whether the amount of constrictor produced is more or less in the body? Certainly, one can hypothesize if this occurs in the experiments using a laboratory environment, this certainly could also lead to an analogous result in the human body.

Even with all the experiments of machines, constrictors, and chlorides having been performed, the blood pressure measuring certainly still cannot be done in the test tube. However, this gives no reason for us to suspect the role chloride and its role in hypertension is impossible and not true.

Thus the question to be asked is could the presence of chloride in the human body decide whether the amount of constrictor produced is more or less in the body?

Certainly it can. It can be explained from the following example. In our life, machines are employed to make consumer products. In other words, for a product to be made, a machine is required. Generally, a commercial machine requires electric power to perform the work. Without electricity (juice), the machine cannot perform the work. For example, an electric saw can cut the wood. Without electric supply, the saw can't function to cut wood. A powerful electric saw cut wood faster, and therefore, more pieces of wood will be cut. The greater the amount of power, the more work being performed and thus also results to more products on market.

We have already mentioned above that there is a lot of so-called equivalent to "machines" in the human body making various products. However, human machines require an analogous type of electricity too. Constrictors are one of the products being made by the machine. As an analogy to the saw example above, the electricity here is called "cofactor" in biochemistry. The cofactor (electric) here will be defined as chloride and is required for producing constrictors. The amount of constrictor produced is dependent more or less on the amount of this electric (chloride).

The greater the amount of chloride, the greater the amount of constrictor (ang II) formed by the "machine"—the ACE (Cushman and Cheung 1971). This was already documented in test-tube studies. Chloride is the required juice (electricity) for this specific machine. The greater the amount of chloride present, the more constrictors could be produced. Thus it would result in increased constriction of the blood vessels, and as discussed above, the blood pressure rises. And as a result, the systolic pressure would also be found higher.

Let's assume that there is no electricity and no chloride in the body. Obviously, there would be a decrease in the amount of formation of constrictors (Cushman and Cheung 1971). As a result, there would be little constriction of the vessels and, very likely, no increase in blood pressure.

From the above explanations, the role of chloride is certainly a factor in deciding the amount of constrictor produced in the human body.

We have discussed a lot related to the role of sodium chloride. The role of sodium-controlled water retention and diastolic pressure is quite clear. Chloride related to the constriction and systolic pressure is also clear in theory.

However, for proving this suggested theory, you will find it from the following.

Sodium chloride is more than likely part of anyone's daily diet. I though I would share my own personal experiences with respect to the consumption of sodium chloride, medicines, and hypertension. As discussed above, these are my own experiences and opinions and should not be a substitute for discussing your health concerns and issues with your own personal doctor.

Personal Experiences

I have a history with high blood pressure beginning around 1987. In 1984, my blood pressure was considered normal (110/72). In 1987, I was beginning to have a slight high blood pressure around 132/92. Gradually, my blood pressure increased year after year. The highest blood pressure obtained during that period was 164/104. I have tried all kind of medications from the medical center at my place of employment. The best pressures observed with medication were lowered to the average 132/92, but despite trying various alternatives, it couldn't be decreased. I understand this situation occurs in many patients.

After I retired, my family doctor tried so hard to lower my blood pressure to normal levels through medication. This was not achieved again.

Thus, with the cooperation of my family doctor and during the beginning of this process, we started trying various blood pressure-lowering drugs. Some were even invented, specifically, in our group by my employer, such as Capoten and Monopril. Before we started this experiment, my blood pressure was about 140/99. After the medication started, my blood pressure dropped to 130/90 and couldn't be dropped any further. This situation was just as what had occurred before I retired; my blood pressure was also decreased to the values of about 132/92 at that time. Thus there must be some reason why this slightly higher blood pressure can't be further decreased to a more normal level.

Under this circumstance, I decided to eliminate sodium chloride from my meals. The method to remove salt would be talked a little later in the next page.

Surprisingly, about two to three weeks later, I felt very uncomfortable and terribly dizzy. I tried to figure out why I was so dizzy. I surmised that my blood pressure might be too low. This was confirmed when I measured my blood pressure immediately and found out that it was indeed low—as low as 90/57, systolic and diastolic pressures, respectively.

In the past, my blood pressure was in no such way lowered to such levels for more than fifteen years. Now it only required two to three weeks time for my blood pressure to the low blood pressure range if I consciously cut out salt. This was unbelievable to me.

Well, feeling dizzy is not how one wants to live through life; therefore, it took me roughly about one year until I found a way to bring the blood pressure back to normal. The way to bring the blood pressure back to normal is by eating with a controlled amount of sodium chloride adjusted daily by a monitor.

However, even though we generally talk about removing sodium chloride from our diet by removing the addition of salt, there is still some amount of sodium chloride present in our food naturally. This internal salt should be removed too. It can be removed also. How? As an example, immerse the food in a continually boiling water for several minutes, then pour the boiling water away and repeat this process two more times. Not only does this process remove the salt, but other salts, oil, lipid, sugars, and other ingredients will also be removed in this process. After two to three weeks of this dietary process, my blood pressure, which averaged 130/90, dropped further down to a much lower pressure range such as 90/57. In the past, I was not able to drop the blood pressure in any way. Now the blood pressure can be dropped and only requires a very short period of time of two to three weeks. Even with drug treatment, generally, it is difficult to drop the blood pressure to such a significantly lower range for any individual. Thus it can be seen how powerful the sodium chloride salt contributes to hypertension. Therefore controlling the amount of sodium chloride diet, under the direction of your doctor, can be one of the best methods to lower high blood pressure.

Later, I tried this similar experiment again and wanted to further prove these results can be reproduced.

I tried to add sodium chloride back to the diet in one or two meals only. My blood pressure was raised to average 140/95 immediately in the next day or two. Then several days later, it returned back to the normal level or even lower after I removed sodium chloride from my diet again. I tried many times, sometimes even with longer period with intake of sodium chloride for two to three weeks. And the identical results would be observed each time. I tried it again for several days, weeks, a month, several months, half a year, one year, and several years later. The same result occurred when I removed salt from the diet.

From these findings, since then, I can control my blood pressure well without any problem.

Sometimes hypertension may be derived from a condition of two different kinds of salts (sodium salt and chloride salt together). Sodium salt and chloride salt together is the sodium chloride single compound in the body resulting to the identical condition of hypertension occurring. Thus sodium chloride salt is still considered as the one to cause hypertension and not the two different salts because both conditions have identical situations of sodium and chloride present together.

After this finding, my family doctor mentioned that, together, we have learned a lot from this "experiment" that will assist him in dealing with patients with high blood pressure.

Volunteers

A.   A friend of mine talked to me about her father in Taiwan with high blood pressure, which wasn't being controlled well under the physician's care. After my suggestions, she called her father and told him to take food with a decreased intake of sodium chloride or only tiny amount of sodium chloride.

Several months later, she happily told me that her father's blood pressure was also under control.

B.   Another friend of mine worked in the same pharmaceutical company with me but in a different department. We have more than forty years of friendship. One day, his wife told me that she felt quite uncomfortable with headaches because of high blood pressure even though she has been taking high blood pressure medication, the drug treatment prescribed by her family doctor for many years.

After my friend and his wife listened to my theory and explanation, as I described above, she said she would try my suggestion. However, after I had visited them three more times within the last two and a half years, she still hadn't proactively attempted to reduce her sodium chloride intake, and her blood pressure remained high. In my last visit, she told me that she will try it this time but has to wait until the upcoming several dinner parties were finished.

Several months later, she told me, "I have a very good news for you." After trying my suggestion, she felt very comfortable, and her blood pressure was in good shape.

She went to her family doctor's office. Her family doctor was also surprised and asked her, "What happened to you? Your blood pressure is fine now." Her answer was that nothing happened except, even though she still took the doctor's prescribed medicine, she didn't exactly follow the doctor's way, but reduced her salt intake.

C. On the evening of February 20, 2008, a friend called me and told me that he and his colleagues went to a conference. They stayed overnight in the hotel and had dinner in a restaurant. They all drank a bowl of soup. Afterward, all of them drank a lot of water because they were too thirsty. After returning to the hotel, they tried measuring their blood pressures. All of them were so afraid because they found their blood pressure to be too high. My friend indicated his systolic value was 170.

From the above personal evidence and a few volunteers, from the author's view, these results are extremely important. It is the author's hope that this information can help you control your high blood pressure, but please discuss any changes under the direction of your physician.

Trying to lower your blood pressure, in general, means lowering both your systolic and diastolic pressures unless one of these values is abnormal. With your doctor's supervision, you should reduce the sodium chloride salt in your diet. It is also one of the simplest methods in lowering your blood pressure. Otherwise, drug treatment may be required. Sometimes, even with drug treatment, it cannot be appropriately reduced.

Therefore, what can be concluded from the above?

A. For hypertension from a diet standpoint, we have the following: Sodium chloride (table salt) is the real cause of high blood pressure.

   1. Sodium plays a role in the retention of water to increase the blood volume in the heart, thereby resulting in the rise of the diastolic pressure in the relaxation step of the heartbeat.

2. Chloride plays a role in constriction (vasoconstriction) and causes the blood vessels to become harder and the size of the opening of the vessels to become smaller, thus resulting to the systolic pressure being higher in the contraction step of the same heartbeat.

B. From a medication and personal point of view and subject to the close care of your physician, we have the following:

1. If the diastolic blood pressure is high, a diuretic drug such as HCTZ (hydrochlorothiazide) should be used to lower the blood pressure.
2. If the systolic blood pressure is higher, either drugs of ACE inhibitor such as Capoten or AII receptor antagonist such as Cozaar should be used to lower the blood pressure.
3. If both the systolic and diastolic pressures are higher, mixed drugs of ACE inhibitor and diuretic agents such as Monopril and HCTZ or AII receptor antagonist and diuretic agents such as Cozaar and HCTZ, combined together, should be used as cocktail therapy to lower this kind of high blood pressure.
4. If the blood pressure is higher due to a higher heartbeat, a βB (beta-blocker) should be used to lower the heartbeat rate and blood pressure.
5. If the blood pressure is higher due to higher cholesterol level, then cholesterol drugs such as Lipitol must be used. It does not just lower cholesterol level and blood pressure, but also helps prevent the occurrence of heart attack and stroke.

C. If you follow the above concept, try the following:

1. Watch your daily diet with intake of a decreased (correct) amount of sodium chloride based on the monitoring of your blood pressure daily to control the intake amount of sodium chloride. Your blood pressure should be under control and may even require no further medication (before you discontinue the use of any medication, please consult with your physician).

Hypotension

We are aware of the causes of high or low blood pressure related to sodium chloride presence in the body. It is a good time to talk a little about the *hypo*tension (low blood pressure) here.

The cause of low blood pressure can be simply stated as not enough blood in the heart. The reason of not having enough blood in the heart is due to the low amount (volume) of blood in the heart and, therefore, results to lower blood pressure. As mentioned above, the more the amount of blood volume in the heart, the higher the blood pressure. Whereas lower blood volume in the heart means lower blood pressure would occur.

The cause of low blood amount or volume in the heart is not enough amount of water in the heart, and it is also due to not enough sodium chloride in the body.

It is very clear to us from the above discussions that either an increased or decreased amount, more or less, of sodium chloride presence is the direct cause of increased or decreased blood pressure. It is because of the presence of the sodium component in sodium chloride having the strong ability to absorb water. Therefore, consuming more of sodium chloride will result in more water being absorbed by the sodium that enters the heart and blood vessels. Thus the amount of blood volume would certainly be increased in the vessels and heart. Especially in the heart, the amount or volume of blood, if it is increased, will result in the blood pressure automatically being increased. This raised blood pressure in the heart is related to the diastolic pressure.

Simultaneously, the part of chloride from eating more sodium chloride would promote more constrictors produced. Thus, as discussed above, the increased amount of constrictors will constrict the vessel harder and result in an increased blood pressure. This increased blood pressure is related to the systolic pressure.

Under this condition, both systolic and diastolic pressures would be increased simultaneously by eating more sodium chloride in meals. Certainly, it could help alleviate the condition of hypotension.

Conclusion

We can say that hypertension and hypotension are both results of the dietary intake of sodium chloride salt. Thus, if the diet of sodium chloride can be controlled, more than likely, both hypertension and hypotension also can be under control.

However, trying to control sodium chloride salt in our diet is very hard and not that easy. Who is willing to change their lifestyle and eating habits such as not smoking, drinking, or reducing salt in food? Some people will still insist to do it. However, when one eats in restaurants, the amount of salt cannot be closely monitored and controlled. Thus one's habits is likely hard to achieve, and treatment by drugs will most likely be needed for one's entire lifetime.

Pressures, blood pressures, and on why blood pressures are high and what substances cause hypertension are all mentioned above. However, how we cure hypertension is not yet mentioned, except by reducing the consumption of sodium chloride.

Drug treatment is also briefly mentioned in section B of this chapter. The concept for the drug treatment will be discussed in the next chapter.

Chapter 6

Medication of High Blood Pressure

The following is a list of the names of the drugs used in treating high blood pressure in alphabetical order. These drugs will also be listed alphabetically in another table referred to as categories of hypertension drugs. The different names of the drugs will also be listed in the third table.

Names of Drugs

Please see the table below. All the names of drugs here are from Health Square. Please see the Web site http://www.healthsquare.com/nav_indices/hbp_index2.htm.

Drugs for hypertension (1)

Names of Drugs (Hypertension)		
Accupril	Bisoprolol	Diovan
Accuretic	with HCTZ	Diuril
Acebutolol	Calan	Doxazosin
Aceon	Candesartan Cilexetil	Dyazide
Adalat	with HCTZ	Enalapril
Aldactazide	Capoten	Enalapril
Aldactone	Capozide	with Felodipine
Aldomet	Captopril	Enalapril
AtlSace	with HCTZ	with HCTZ

Amiloride with HCTZ	Captopril	Esidrix
	Cardene	Felodipine
Amlodipine	Cardizen	Fosinopril (Monopril)
	Cardura	Furosemide
Amlodipine with Benazepril	Carvedilol	Guanfacine Hydrochloride
Atacand HCT	Catapres	Hydrochlorothiazide
Atacand	Chlorothiazide	Hydrochlorothiazide with Triamterene
Atenolol	Chlothialidone	
Atenolol with Chlorthalidone	Clonidine	HydroDIURIL
	Coreg	Hytrin
Avalide	Cogard (Nadolol)	Hyzaar
Avapro	Cozide	Indapamide
Benazepril	Covera-HS	Inderal
Benazepril with HCTZ	Cozaar	Inderide
	Demadex	Irbesartan (Avapro)
Benicar	Dilacor XR	Isoptin
Bisoprolol	Diltizen	Isradipine

Drugs for hypertension (2)

Names of Drugs (Hypertension)		
Labetalol	Nadolol with	Tenoretic
Lasix	Bendroflumethiazide	Tenomin
Lexxel	Nicardipine	Terazosin
Lisinopril	Nifedipine	Teveten
Lisinopril with HCTZ	Nisoldipine	Teveten HCT
Lopressor	Nomodyne	Thailtone
Losartan with HCTZ	Norvasc	Tiazac
Lotensin HCT	Pintolol	Toprol-XL
Lotensin	Plendil	Torsemide
Lotrel	Prazosin	Trandate
Lozol	Prinivil	Trandolapril
Marvik	Prinzide	Trandolapril with verapamil
Maxzide	Procardia	Uniretic
Methyldopa	Propranolol	Univasc
Metolazone	Propranolol with HCTZ	Valsartan
Metoprolol	Quinapril	Vaseretic
Micardis	Ramipril	Vasotec (Enalapril)
Minipress	Sectral	Verapamil
Moduretic	Spironolactone	Verelan
Moexpril	Spironolactone with HCTZ	Zaoxolyn
Moexpril with HCTZ	Sular	Zebeta
Mykrox	Tarka	Zestoretic
Nadolol	Telmisartan	Zestril
	Telmisartan with HCTZ	Ziac

The above drugs will also be relisted in this table as a category, making it is easy for the readers to know what kind of function the drug is related to.

In the following table, the abbreviations in the left column are spelled out in the right column.

1.	ACEI	ACE(angiotensin-converting enzyme inhibitor)
2.	ACEI + Ca^{++} CB	ACE inhibitor + Calcium Channel Blocker
3.	ACEI + D	ACE inhibitor + Diuretic agent
4.	AII RA	AII (angiotensin II) receptor antagonist
5.	AII RA + D	AII receptor antagonist + Diuretic agent
6.	D	Diuretic agent (Water pill)
7.	Ca^{++} CB	Calcium channel blocker
8.	βB	Beta-blocker
9.	βB + D	Beta-blocker + Diuretic agent
10.	αB	Alpha-blocker

Categories of hypertensive Drugs (1)

ACEI	ACEI + Ca++CB	ACEI + D	AII RA
Accupril		Accuretic	Atacand
Aceon	Amlodipine, Benazepril	benazepril, HCTZ	Avapro
Altace		Capozide	Benicar
Benazepril	Enalapril, Felodipine	Captopril, HCTZ	Cozaar
Capoten	Lexxel	Enalapril, HCTZ	Diovan
Captopril	Lotrel	Lisinopril, HCTZ	Irbesartan
Enalapril	Tarka	Lotensin HCT	Losartan
Fosinopril	Trandolapril, verapamil	Moexpril, HCTZ	Micardis
Lisinopril		Prinzide	Telmisartan
Lotensin		Quinapril, HCTZ	Teveten
Marvik		Uniretic	Valsartan
Moexpril		Zestoretic	
Monopril			
Prinivil			
Quinapril			
Ramipril			
Trandolapril			
Univasc			
Vaseretic			
Vasotec			
Zestril			

Categories of hypertensive Drugs (2)

AII RA + D	D	Ca⁺⁺ CB
Avalide	Aldactazide	Adalat
Candesartan, HCTZ	Aldactone	Amlodipine
	Amiloride,HCTZ	Calan
Hyzaar	Chlorothiazide	Cardene
Micardis	Chlothialidone	Cardizen
Teveten HCT	Demadex	Covera-HS
Atacand HCT	Diuril	Dilacor XR
Losartan, HCTZ	Dyazide	Diltizen
Micardis HCTZ	Esidrix	Felodipine
Telmisartan, HCTZ	Furosemide	Isoptin
	HCTZ + Triamterene	Isradipine
	HCTZ	Nicardipine
	HydroDIURIL	Nifedipine
	Indapamide	Nisoldipine
	Lasix	Norvasc
	Lozol	Plendil
	Maxzide	Procardia
	Metolazone	Sular
	Moduretic	Tiazac
	Mykrox	Verapamil
	Spironolactone,HCTZ	Verelan
	Spironolactone	
	Thailtone	
	Torsemide	
	Zaroxolyn	

Categories of hypertensive Drugs (3)

βB	βB + D	αB	Others
Acebutolol	Atenolol, Chlorthalidone	Cardura	Aldomet
Atenolol	Bisoprolol With HCTZ	Hytrin	Cardura
Bisoprolol	Corzide	Minipress	Carvedilol
Cogard	Nadolol with Bendroflumethiazide	Prazosin	Catapres
Coreg		Terazosin	Doxazosin
Guanfacine HCl	Propranolol with HCTZ		Labetalol
Inderal	Ziac		Methyldopa
Lopressor			Nomodyne
Metoprolol			Trandate
Nadolol			
Pindolol			
Propanolol			
Sectral			
Tenormin			
Toprol-XL			
Zebeta			

In general, the drug in each group is used to treat the hypertension as follows:

1. ACEI   To shut off the machine, then to block the constrictor formation, and to prevent the vessel harder **to lower the systolic blood pressure**. (In some patients, coughing and itching would occur. However, by switching to AII RA drugs, this symptom will be disappeared. Effect to the disease is identical.)

2. ACEI + Ca^{++} CB   Combines the effects of ACEI and Ca^{++} CB to lower blood pressures.

3. ACEI + D   Combines the effects of ACEI and D. It can **lower both systolic and diastolic pressures very effectively**.

4. AII RA   To block the constrictor entering from his office to work. There is no constriction of the vessel. It prevents the vessel from getting harder, resulting **to lower systolic pressure**.

5. AII RA + D   Combines both the effects of AII RA and D. It can **lower both systolic and diastolic pressures very effectively**.

6. D   To remove water from human body (specifically from the heart) leading **to lower diastolic pressure**. Precaution: the potassium level could be low.

7. Ca^{++} CB   Calcium channel blocker is also **observed to have the function of decreasing the heart pumping rate.**

8. βB   **Reduces the heart's pumping rate (beat) to lower blood pressure.**

9. βB + D   Combines both the effects of βB and D to lower blood pressure.

10. βB   Increases the urination **rate to remove water to lower blood pressure.**

Drugs with different names are listed in this table.

Drugs with different names (1)

Accupril	=	Quinapril	Corgard	=	Nadolol
Accuretic	=	Quinapril with HCTZ	Corzide	=	Nadolol with Bendroflumethiazide
Acebutolol	=	Sectral			
Adalate	=	Procardia	Cozaar	=	Losartan
Aldactazide	=	Spinonolactone HCTZ	Demadex	=	Torsemide
Aldactone	=	Spironolactone	Diovan	=	Valsartan
Aldomet	=	Methyldopa	Diuril	=	Chlorothiazide
Altace	=	Ramipril	Dyazide	=	Maxzide
Atacand	=	Candesdesartan Cilexetil	Felodipine	=	Plendil
			Fosinopril	=	Monopril
Atacand HCT	=	Candesdesartan Cilexetil HCT	Hydrochlorothiazide = HCTZ		
			HydroDiuril	=	HCTZ
Avapro	=	Irbesartan	Hytrin	=	Terazosin
Avaslide	=	Irbesartan HCTZ	Hyzaar	=	Losartan, Cozaar, with HCTZ
Bisoprolo	=	Zebeta			
Bisoprolo HCTZ	=	Ziac	Inderal	=	Propranolol
Calan	=	Verapamil, Covera-HS, Isoptin, Verelan	Inderide	=	Propranolol + HCTZ
Capoten	=	Captopril	Labetalol	=	Normodyne, Trandate
Capozide	=	Captopril HCTZ			
			Lasix	=	Furosemide
Cardene	=	Nicardipine	Lexxel	=	Enalapril with Felodipine
Cardizem	=	Dilacor XR, Tiazac			
Cardura	=	Doxazosin	Lisinopril	=	Zestril, Prinivil
Catapres	=	Clonidine	Lopressor	=	Toprol, Metoprolol
Coreg	=	Carvedilol	Lotensin	=	Benazepril

Drugs with different names (2)

Lotensin HCT	=	Benazepril HCT	Prinzide	=	Zestoretic, Lisinopril HCTZ
Lotrel	=	Amlodipine Benazepril	Procardia	=	Nifedipine
Lozol	=	Indapamide			
Mavik	=	Trandolapril	Tarka	=	Varapamil, Trandolapril
Metolazone	=	Zaroxolyn			
Micardis	=	Telmisartan	Tenormin	=	Atenolol
Micardis HCT	=	Telmisartan with HCTZ	Tenoretic	=	Atenolol with Chlorthiazide
Minipress	=	Prazosin	Thalitone	=	Chlorthalidone
Moduretic	=	Amiloide HCTZ	Uniretic	=	Moexipril with HCTZ
Mykrox	=	Zaroxolyn	Univasc	=	Moexipril
Nisoldipine	=	Sular	Vaseretic	=	Enalapril with HCTZ
Norvasc	=	Amlodipine	Vasotec	=	Enalapril

To cure high blood pressure, only two kinds of blood pressure—systolic and diastolic pressures—should be of concern. It could be for either one or for both. Thus, totally, three conditions (systolic pressure high, diastolic pressure high, or both pressures high) could happen. Even if the three conditions happen, only two different blood pressures could be high. For this reason, lowering high blood pressure requires lowering either high systolic pressure or high diastolic pressure or both.

1.　Cause of High Systolic Pressure

Function

High systolic pressure is a result of increased amounts of constrictor produced in the human body by the chloride, which then leads to the function of constricting the vessels such that they are harder and then causing the diameter of vessels to become smaller. Thus systolic pressure is increased.

If there are no constrictors produced in the body, the vessels will not increase its constriction, and as a result, the blood pressure should not be elevated.

Diet (Sodium Chloride)

The part of one's daily diet that can cause systolic pressure to rise is the intake of chloride. Chloride is part of sodium chloride. Therefore, if there is no sodium chloride in the human body, fewer constrictors will be produced, and hypertension will not likely occur. The high systolic pressure will also be lowered too. Thus the intake of less or a minimal amount of sodium chloride should result to the high systolic pressure returning back to normal or even lower.

2.　Cause of High Diastolic Pressure

Function

A high diastolic pressure is the result of water overloading in the body by sodium and then induces too much water into the heart and the vessels. The increased amount of water in the heart results to more blood in the heart. The increased amount of blood in the heart certainly causes the diastolic pressure to be too high.

To lower the high diastolic pressure, the blood volume in the heart must be dropped. After the water is removed, the high diastolic pressure should lower automatically.

Diet (Sodium Chloride)

As discussed above for systolic pressure, the part of one's daily diet that can cause the systolic pressure to rise is the intake of chloride. However, the other cause is sodium. Sodium is part of sodium chloride. Therefore, if there is no sodium chloride in the human body, less water will be absorbed in the body; and hypertension will not likely occur. The higher diastolic pressure will also be lowered too. Thus the intake of less or a minimal amount of sodium chloride should result to the high diastolic pressure returning back to normal or even lower

Then with minimal salt in the diet, both high systolic and diastolic pressures would be lowered simultaneously and return back to normal or even lower pressures.

3.   *Concept of Hypertension Treatment*

Medications/drugs

a.   *Lower the high systolic pressure.*

The ACE inhibitor (ACEI) or AII receptor antagonist (AII RA) can be used for this kind of treatment. Please refer to the item of drug category in this chapter.

b.   *Lower the high diastolic pressure.*

Diuretic (D) drug can be used for this kind of treatment. Please refer also to the item of drug category in this chapter.

c. *Lower both high systolic and diastolic pressures simultaneously.*

Combination of ACE inhibitor (ACEI) and diuretic (D) drugs or combination of AII receptor antagonist (AII RA) and diuretic (D) drugs can be used simultaneously to lower both high blood pressures. Please refer also to the item of drug category in this chapter.

d. *Lower high blood pressure is from the fast heart rate.*

To lower this kind of high blood pressure, drugs for lowering the heart rate can be used such as beta-blocker (βB). Please refer also to the item of drug category in this chapter.

e. *Higher blood pressure is from too much cholesterol in the blood.*

Drugs used to lower the cholesterol such as Lipitor can be used to lower this kind of high blood pressure. A cholesterol-lowering drug is not a blood pressure-lowering drug. Thus it is not related to the subject in this book.

As discussed above, this should be used simply as a reference to know your hypertension condition. None of these recommendations above should be taken unless you have the approval of your doctor.

Diet.

Just reduced or controlled the only diet of sodium chloride, both situations of hypertension, systolic and/or diastolic pressures would certainly be lowered too.

Even this method is very simple, however do you think you can do it. This is the question.

All above, just as reference you should talk with doctor.

Chapter 7

Other Thoughts

It is a good idea to discuss some other issues related to health, illness, and drugs.

Congestive Heart Failure

Congestive heart failure is a disease resulting from hypertension. Its cause: the heart can't pump all the amount of blood out to the artery. There are small amounts of blood still remaining in the heart chamber after each pump (contraction step). The question is why does the small amount of blood remain in the heart chamber after each pump (contraction cycle)? Usually, it occurs as the heart weakens.

Remember, the average heartbeat is 75 beats per minute. Each beat, *on the average,* requires *0.8 second (60 sec / 75 beats = 0.8 sec per beat).* There are two different cycles or steps (contraction and relaxation) in each one beat (pulse). Each single step requires half the time for one beat. Thus the time required for each single step is half of the 0.8 seconds. It is 0.4 seconds (0.8 sec / 2 = 0.4 sec). The contraction cycle must complete the job of pumping and pushing all the blood out to the artery in this limited short period of time—0.4 sec, and a huge force must be required to complete this work. In case the force or energy is not strong enough, this work cannot be accomplished, and there will be some amount of blood remaining in the heart chamber after each beat.

The normal pressure average is 115/75. As mentioned in the previous chapter, 115 is systolic pressure value. It is a pressure powerful enough to pump all blood out from heart to the artery. The diastolic pressure value is 75. It is heart's basic control pressure and the pressure in which blood could remain in the heart. As mentioned before, the more the amount of blood in heart, the higher the diastolic pressure will be. How high the value of diastolic pressure will depend on how much more blood there is in the heart. Therefore, the higher or lower diastolic pressure is strictly dependent on the amount of blood, more or less, present in the heart.

In the event the normal diastolic pressure is 75, it is also the pressure of blood remaining in the heart. Under this condition, for all blood to be pushed out completely in such a short time frame of 0.4 second, a strong force is required. Definitely it must be much higher than the diastolic pressure of 75. Under this circumstance, the heart's 115 systolic pressure pushes its 75 diastolic pressure. In this condition, the heart's 115 systolic pressure should be powerful enough to enable all blood to be pushed out from the heart into the artery, and no more blood would remain in the heart.

The normal systolic pressure is 115. If the pushing force (systolic pressure) changed and dropped to 75, it is just equal to the normal diastolic pressure. Thus the pushing force (systolic pressure) 75 and the heart's basic (diastolic) force 75 is equal to each other. Thus no blood can be pushed out from the heart into the artery in this manner.

Only when the pushing force is much higher than the diastolic pressure 75 will the blood be pushed out, but not necessary all will be pushed out under this condition.

And only under this occurrence **can the normal pushing force (systolic pressure) be 115**. It is about 53% higher than the diastolic pressure (115/75 = 153.3% or 153%). Under this normal condition, the systolic pressure requires 53% more on top of the diastolic pressure of 75 to accomplish this work. When the systolic pressure is 115, it is powerful enough to push the diastolic pressure of 75, and all the blood, therefore, would be found to be pushed completely out from the heart into the artery in the short time of 0.4 sec. Also, no amount of blood would remain in the heart.

If the pushing force is less than 115 (e.g., 100) and the diastolic pressure is still 75, the blood can be pushed out, but can't be completely pushed out in this fashion in such a short period of time of 0.4 sec, and therefore, a small amount of blood would be found remaining in the heart after this pumping.

The above explanation indicates how congestive heart failure could occur and also why an amount of blood may still be found remaining in the heart chamber after each pumping action (pulse). However this example above may not be what is occurring for congestive heart failure as explained below.

What happens? The greater the amount of blood found in the heart will result in the diastolic pressure being found to be higher also. It may reach values of 100 (example) or even higher. Under this circumstance, assuming the normal systolic pressure is still at 115, certainly this pressure with a pushing force of 115 may be not stronger enough for the higher diastolic pressure, such as 100 or higher, for the job of pushing. After this pumping action, some amount of blood must be found remaining in the heart. A pushing force (systolic pressure) of 115 is good enough for a diastolic pressure of 75 and definitely not necessarily strong enough for a diastolic pressure 100 or even higher. Under this condition, of course, a partial amount of blood could possibly remain in the heart after each heartbeat.

Even the systolic pressure could be readjusted automatically to the higher values in the body and matched up with the higher diastolic pressure value. Still, this readjustment step for higher systolic pressure values occuring in the body may not be strong enough, and therefore, it is not necessarily good enough to match and reach the required pushing force, the systolic pressure values. Thus this work still can't be performed in this situation. Some amounts of blood may still remain in the heart after this pumping action. Congestive heart failure, thus, would still occur under this condition.

Usually, congestive heart failure may occur from an excessive intake of sodium chloride in the diet. To treat the congestive heart failure, the medicine will help but not very effectively. However, if the total amount of blood can be controlled in the heart, the congestive heart failure will automatically disappear even without drug treatment.

A question to be answered is how could the total amount of blood be controlled in the heart? To do it, an increased amount of blood should never be allowed to be present in the heart. As discussed above, the increased amount of blood is due to more water found in the heart. The more the water presence, also leads to the conclusion of an increased total amount of blood in the heart.

As discussed above, an increased amount of water occurring in the heart is the result of an increased intake of sodium chloride. Sodium in sodium chloride contributes the strong ability to absorb a large amount of water with sodium chloride that is present in the body. Thus it leads to the water, and therefore, an increase in blood volume in the heart. As a result, the diastolic pressure is much higher and can lead to potential congestive heart failure.

In case the intake amount of sodium chloride is dropped in the body, the water and blood volume will be automatically reduced to the normal level. Thus the risk for the disease of congestive heart failure will be reduced automatically.

Diseases Always Happen to Everybody

There are so many different diseases. To understand and treat the diseases is not simple at all. One always wonders whether these diseases are curable or not.

In general, some can be cured with medications and not require further medications after being cured. However, some require medications for their whole life to control that disease.

How can we know which kind of disease is curable and does not require continuous medication?

In general, there are two major kinds of diseases that can be discussed.

1. Resulting from Outside Influences

These diseases can result from injuries such as being cut, from virus or bacteria, and so on. These illnesses are results of external influences. In such illnesses, no more medications or medical treatment are further required after being cured.

We can use following example to explain it.

If you have a problem with your car, you will get your problem fixed in the garage or with a car dealer. With you or me, if we have a medical issue, we will see a doctor to take care of our issue.

If the battery on the car is bad, the engine can't be started at all. However, after the battery is replaced, the engine will start immediately. No further fixing is required.

In a car, the replacement of parts to fix the problem is from an external cause to the engine. For an illness to you and me, this could also result from an external cause and then to the body. Such kind of illnesses after being cured (such as bacteria and virus as described above) will result in, hopefully, no further medication and medical attention.

2. Resulting from Internal Influences

Using the car example, if the battery is replaced and the engine can't be started, the problem may not be from the bad battery.

Perhaps the car is out of gas. The only way, then, to start the engine is to refuel the car. After refueling, the engine will start immediately. The engine will shut down again when the gas is all gone. Therefore, the car will require the refueling of gas to run the engine for its life.

For you or me, if the illness occurs internally in human body, we need to refuel with some necessary requirements to human organs and body just as refueling gas to the engine of a car. Therefore, illnesses can occur from related changed items in the body such as a diabetic with too much sugar and unable to process such sugar appropriately.

Drugs Are Always Found to Have Side Effects

Are there any drugs that doesn't have a side effect? Treatment using drugs always has listed side effects. However, let's discuss the situation when the occurrence of the side effect is not because of the drug but rather from the **dose** (amount) of the drug used.

In the human body, side effects always occur. It happens not just through the intake of the drug, but also occurs in other areas. As an example, if one drinks too much water, one will feel uncomfortable. If one eats too much, then the resulting side effect is to feel uncomfortable and bloated.

In our environment, too much rain will result in flooding. Too much snow can result in many accidents on the road. These are also examples of side effects of excessive amounts in our environment. These analogies also apply to our bodies.

If we are aware of all these, we will realize from these examples, that the side effect is not from the drug, but rather is a result of the overdose (amount).

As a result, a lesser amount may reduce the side effect. However, one needs to be careful in reducing any amount prescribed by their doctor; it may not be effective enough for disease treatment. Therefore, please consult with your doctor.

In addition to drugs, anything in our body, if excessive, can result to a related side effect such as illnesses occurring. Generally, a lesser amount will reduce the side effect. The side effect occurring is not just related to the amount in the body, but if any biological thing such as air or sugar or if any missing or new thing such as virus or bacteria is found in the body, it will certainly also result to a related side effect and, hence, an illness occurring in the body. Cancer is an example where too many adverse cells are occurring. Thus the side effect could be considered as a disease.

How Can Diseases Develop Internally?

As mentioned earlier in this chapter, one of the illnesses occurring results internally. First we have to understand why do diseases occur within us.

We have to understand that there are many things in the human body. All things are chemicals and required, thus called biochemicals, such as sodium chloride salt, sugar, oil, cholesterol, and others. All things in the human body are required substances. They must be present but must be in a correct amount (normal level) in the body.

The amount (level) of everything distributed in each organ and tissue in the human body is different. However, each of them must be kept in the correct amount (right level) in each part of the body and must also be matched with the ages. In case (1) any is missing or (2) newly found or (3) the amount can't be controlled (changed to either high or low or low to high) in the body, a related illness will occur within the body. It is also a side effect. For example, too much sugar (amount) in the body can result to diabetes. Too much cholesterol (amount) in the body can result to a heart attack. An influx of harmful or excessive bacteria and virus (new) in the system can result to an infection and/or illness. Without air (missing), humans could die.

All items' presence and amount are maintained in the human body must be from some sources provided from outside of our body by refueling. A major source of supply is the intake of food. Generally, the intake of food can also be a major source in affecting diseases, which are related to (1) an amount unbalance, (2) control of every item lost (as mentioned above), and (3) new things found inside our body.

To fix this problem, we have to pay attention to (1) the correct (right) amount (right level) of intake, and it must be maintained in the body all the time; (2) no new thing found; and (3) nothing missing in the body. If you can do this, an element affecting the illness can be removed, and the risk of disease can be lowered.

To do this, you must refuel the supply of your body just as you refuel the gas to the engine in a car. If you refuel diesel to your gas engine, the gas engine will not start. So you must refuel with the right gas and not diesel. Thus you must eat the right food (everything) in your meal but remember not to consume an excessive amount. Otherwise, you may need to be prescribed with medication to control the diseases, which may crop up later in your life.

As mentioned above, hypertension is one of the illnesses known from certain things—the amount lost controlled and the balance not maintained. Sodium chloride is the one affecting these and high blood pressures. They are (1) constriction resulting from producing more amounts of constrictor (hypertensive agent) and (2) water retention resulting to more water accumulating in the heart. If under control, both of these conditions—the amount of constrictor and water—should be reduced or eliminated in our body. To do this, the amount of sodium chloride must be watched and must be reduced or eliminated in our body. The amount of sodium chloride, if maintained at the correct amount, can result in hypertension being under control and potentially cured. The medication, therefore, may also not be required. However, the correct amount of sodium chloride required in the body must be monitored based on your blood pressure on a daily basis for life. If you can do this, it is an example that this disease, hypertension, can be under control without drug treatment. Otherwise, you have to use medications to control your hypertension for your life.

A suitable food supply for each person is different and, therefore, is very complicated. Thus, what suitable food in food supply is a big question in human health life.

However, in our daily life, we have no idea how to keep any disease and their related thing maintained at right amounts in our body except the illness of hypertension (already described) and congestive heart failure (described). Under this circumstance, because of the lack of idea on how the illness happened, a drug is required to control that disease for a human's life. In this case, drug will become our most required **food source** to eliminate that related diseases happened.

Why Can Drugs Cure a Disease?

With too much sugar or cholesterol in the body, diabetes and heart attack respectively can occur. However, in the case where the sugar and cholesterol level is normal or those levels have returned back to normal, more than likely, the illness does not occur. Thus the resulting illnesses are directly related to those increased or decreased substance levels in the body such as sugar and cholesterol. Therefore, the uncontrolled amount of that substance may result in a related disease. Under controlled amounts, a decreased risk of related disease should occur or the risk may even be completely eliminated.

With medications such as Lipitor being consumed by patients with high cholesterol, the amount of cholesterol should be reduced and reduced back to the normal level. However, without continued medication, the cholesterol level may increase again; and the symptoms reoccur. Thus medications can cure this kind of disease, a direct result from its ability to control the level of cholesterol back to normal in the human body.

This example on cholesterol treatment also applies to other diseases even with cancer patients. If the cancer cell level can be reduced or eliminated to normal levels with appropriate treatment of drugs, hopefully, the cancer is in remission and/or the symptoms have disappeared.

This is the reason why drugs can cure diseases.

Genetic

Newborn babies usually are all healthy and are not sick. **Why?** The answer is very simple. From birth, a blueprint of genetics is within newborn babies: (1) the amount of everything in their bodies is maintained at the correct amount (right level), (2) anything required are all there, and (3) things not required are not in the body. Due to these facts, all are under control. It is the reason why there are a few illnesses found in a newborn baby unless an abnormal situation occurs at birth. In case any change from the above issues occurs in the baby's body, an illness will occur in the newborn baby immediately.

After being born, the baby keeps growing older. During this growing process, the environment surrounding the body inside out is changing every minute. This time the changing process is also affecting the changes of the body. During this time-changing period, to maintain everything—(1) no new thing found, (2) nothing missing, and (3) the correct amount under controlled in the body—is hard. Its maintenance requires some supply sources to fulfill this goal. This supply source must be provided from outside of baby's body. Generally, it is from the food sources. If (1) everything is there, (2) no new thing happens, and (3) the correct amount is maintained in the body, no illness would happen, and human will have a very health long life. These facts are maintained strictly depending on the supply of outside food sources and the amount, more or less. It is just like the situation of refueling gas to the engine. If any of these is missing from supply sources long enough or interrupted in the middle, it will directly influence any related maintenance not under control that's happening in the body. Those suitable sources if not provided correctly from the food supply will directly result to that specific related responsible illness happening. Eating too much oil and fat sources will directly influence the buildup of cholesterol in the body, and the cholesterol level certainly couldn't be maintained. Finally it could threaten one's life to have heart attack.

Thus, those facts maintained are extremely important in the body. However, in our human life, even if we know that those fact are important, we usually ignored it and do not pay attention at all or can't keep it up in our life all the time. Disease certainly developed later.

However, the same food supply sources usually do not apply only to you in your family. They are also for all members of your whole family.

In case the same unsuitable food source supplies last longer enough in your family, the identical developed situation "any one (1) such as missing items, (2) new substance found, or (3) amount cannot be maintained" will happen to the body of everyone in your family. Same disease, thus, will also possibly occur to every member in your family but not to the other families.

Usually, the same disease is commonly found and observed to be occurring in pattern in members of the same family, such as diabetes, hypertension, and so on. These kinds of illnesses are usually referred to as the genetic type. The genetic disease is identical to the illness as discussed herein by the author.

These unbalanced amounts and uncontrolled situations usually occur for long periods of time continuously from the situation of an unsuitable food supply. The side effect and those related responsible illnesses usually occurs and are found by the person later in older age. This is the reason why certain diseases only occur in old age and not in the younger generation.

This situation does not usually occur in the younger generations because this uncontrolled condition could not be developed completely in a short period of time. It is developed gradually and requires a longer period of time. When it develops completely, this situation is usually irreversible. A suitable food supply is no longer able to control the above-mentioned unbalanced amount and uncontrolled situation. It is because many steps would be involved in this long period of change. We don't know which one step is the key factor that caused it. Unless you know which the key factor is, this factor can be controlled by a specific diet. This disease certainly will no longer be there.

Conclusion

An illness is always present, and there is no way to avoid it. It is because the natural environment around us is always changing. The limiting eating habits influence the following conditions: they are (1) the correct amount of everything to be maintained, (2) no new substance found, and (3) nothing missed in the human body. In addition, the knowledge of the illness is still not clear enough.

Hypertension and congestive heart failure are the two diseases known that can be controlled using the concepts in this book. It is by trying to bring the abnormal amount of hypertension related things (internal sodium chloride, table salt) back to normal and kept that way in the body. If you truly do it, after it is under control, medications are no longer required unless we can't totally control our life habits.

One understands illnesses well enough these days. Human knowledge collected on illnesses from the past are now quite extensive. Even the knowledge combined with the above is quite enough but still too far away from understanding. However, everything in nature has a reason. They can all be explained. Unfortunately, due to the limited knowledge, most things can't be explained at this moment for the time being. It definitely can be explained later in the near future or over longer periods of time.

Abbreviations and Meanings

ACE   Angiotensin-converting enzyme

ACEI   ACE (angiotensin converting-enzyme) inhibitor.

ACEI + Ca^{++} CB   ACE inhibitor + Calcium Channel Blocker

ACEI + D   ACE inhibitor + Diuretic agent

AII RA   AII (angiotensin II) recepitor antagonist

AII RA + D   AII receptor antagonist + Diuretic agent

αB   Alpha-blocker

βB   β-blocker, Beta-blocker

βB + D   Beta-blocker + Diuretic agent

Ca^{++} CB   Calcium channel blocker

Chloride   Chloride ion

Constrictor   Angiotensin II

D   Diuretic agent (Water pill)

Dose   Amount

Home station	Receptor
Hypertension	High blood pressure
Juice	Electricity
Machine	Enzyme
Sodium	Sodium ion
Table salt	Sodium chloride

References

Cheung, H.S. 1998, Hypertension and Rational Design of Captopril, the First ACE Inhibitor for the Treatment of Hypertension Kabel Publishers, Rockville, MD,

Cheung, H.S. 2003, Hypertension and Rational Design of Captopril, the First ACE Inhibitor for the Treatment of Hypertension, Kabel Publishers, Rockville, MD,

Chiu, A.T., Carini, D.J., Johnson, A.L., McCall, D.E., Price, W.A., Thoolen, M.J.M.C., Wong, P.C., Taber, R.I. and Timmermans. P.B.M.W.M. 1988. Non-peptide angiotensin II receptor antagonists. II. Pharmacology of S-8308. Eur J Pharmacol 157:13-21

Chiu, A.T., McCall, D.E., Price, W.A., Wong, P.C., Carini, D.J., Duncia, J.V., Wexler, R.R., Yoo, S.E., Johnson, A.L. and Timmermans, P.B.M.W.M. 1990. Nonpeptide angiotensin II receptor antagonist. VII. cellular and biochemical pharmacology of DuP 753, an orally active antihypertensive agent. J Pharmacol Exp Ther 252:711-718

Cushman, D.W. and Cheung, H.S. 1971. Spectrophotometric assay and properties of the angiotensin-converting enzyme of rabbit lung, Biochem Pharmacol 20:1637-1648

Cushman, D.W. and Cheung, H.S. 1972. Studies in vitro of angiotensin-converting enzyme of lung and other tissues. In Hypertension. eds. J. Genest and E. Koiw, pp.532-541, New York: Springer

O'Brien, E. and Fitzgerald, D. 1994. The history of blood pressure measurement. J. Human Hypertension. 8:73-84

Shevchenko, Y.L. and Tsithk, J.E. 1996. 90th anniversary of the development by Niolai S. Korotkoff of the auscultatory method of measuring blood pressure. Circulation 94:116-118

Skeggs, L.T., Marsh, W.H., Kahn, J.R. and Shumway, N.P. 1954. The existence of two forms of hypertensin. J Exp Med 99:275-282

Skeggs, L.T., Kahn, J.R., and Shumway, N.P. 1956. The preparation and function of the hypertension-converting enzyme. J Exp Med 103:295-299

Wong, P.C., Price, W.A., Chiu, A.T., Thoolen, M.J.M.C., Duncia, J.V., Johnson, A.L., and Timmermans, P.B.M.W.M. 1989. Nonpeptide angiotensin II receptor antagonist. IV. EXP6155 and Exp6803. Hypertension 13: 489-497

Index

www.ingramcontent.com/pod-product-compliance
Lightning Source LLC
Chambersburg PA
CBHW031259280526
45784CB00004B/1917

* 9 7 8 1 4 3 6 3 7 8 9 7 0 *